Praise for *Where in the OM Am I?*

"This memoir reads like the best of chick lit, but with far deeper self-reflection....A must-read for yogis (or would-be yogis) who enjoy a little snarkiness with their *savasana*." —*Kirkus Reviews*

"*The Devil Wears Prada* meets *Eat, Pray, Love* in this engaging, inspiring tale of self-discovery. DiVello blends keen cultural observation with a terrifically wry wit as she balances her soul-killing corporate career with the world of New Age poseurs and guru-loving sycophants of her yoga teacher training. A great read for anyone who has ever sat in a cubicle, dreaming of escape."

—Kathleen Flinn, *New York Times* best-selling author of
The Sharper Your Knife, the Less You Cry

"When Sara DiVello tries to fold a yoga practice into her miserable, mirthless corporate career, she realizes even the so-called enlightened aren't immune to back-stabbing bitchery. Raw, real, and at times deeply, darkly funny, *Where in the OM Am I?* shows you a side of yoga you may not have known existed. If you think your job sucks, this book will be more welcome than an extra-long corpse pose at the end of a grueling class."

—Jenna McCarthy, author of *If It Was Easy,
They'd Call the Whole Damn Thing a Honeymoon*

"For the type-A, neurotic, career girl or anyone climbing the corporate ladder and hating it, you need to read this book."

—Beth Orsoff, best-selling author of *Vlad All Over*

Where in the OM Am I?

One Woman's Journey from the Corporate World to the Yoga Mat

Sara DiVello

Worcester Square Press, Boston

Published by Worcester Square Press, Boston, Massachusetts, USA.

Printed in the United States of America.

ISBN: 978-0-9890555-0-5 (pbk.)
ISBN: 978-0-9890555-1-2 (ebk.)

Names and identifying characteristics have been
changed to protect the privacy of certain individuals.

Cover design by Heidi North/Julie Metz, Julie Metz LTD.
Cover illustration by Heidi North.
Original cover photo by Jamie Schulinn.

For Joanie

Authenticity: true to one's own personality, spirit, or character[1]

Chapter Two, Verse 48 in the Bhagavad Gita:

Do your work in the peace of yoga and free from selfish desires,

be not moved in success or in failure....[2]

Chapter Two, Verse 50 in the Bhagavad Gita:

Yoga is skill in action.[3]

Yoga is wisdom in work.[2]

---

[1] *Merriam-Webster Dictionary*, (Enclyclopædia Britannica Company, 2013).

[2] Juan Mascaró, translator, *The Bhagavad Gita* (New York: Penguin Classics, 2003).

[3] Winthrop Sargeant, translator, *The Bhagavad Gita Twenty-Fifth Anniversary Edition* (Albany: State University of New York Press, 2009).

OM ("ॐ" in Sanskrit, the language of yoga): often used at the beginning and end of yoga classes. The sound of OM has been described as all-encompassing, universal in nature.

Author's Note:

This book is a memoir based on my personal experiences working in financial services and attending yoga teacher training. While the characters in this book are based on real people, names and identifying details have been changed to protect privacy, and, in some cases, characters have been combined for the sake of protecting privacy as well as for narrative purposes.

The idea to write a book about my experiences in financial services and yoga only occurred to me after leaving the financial services industry and completing my teacher training. Therefore, I had no occasion to discuss my writing this book with my colleagues, classmates, or yoga-teacher-training instructor at the time of the events depicted herein. For that reason, the events chronicled in this book are unfettered by any influences that the knowledge that someone would write a book about them might otherwise have exerted.

The events I depict in this book are drawn from my memory of those events as well as from my notes and personal journal. I have recreated dialogue from memory and notes, and have in certain instances compressed multiple conversations to capture their substance in a narratively efficient manner. While I consider myself to have an excellent memory, each person's memory of his or her experiences is highly personal and may be imperfect. Therefore, I can only assure you that these were my experiences as I remember them. Other people may have experienced or might recall the same events differently.

Where in the OM Am I?

Prologue: I Once Was Lost...

The day before our one-year anniversary, my then-boyfriend, who had talked openly about imagining us growing old together, surprised me by showing up unannounced at my apartment. Deeply enmeshed in the labyrinth of my first post-college, real-world relationship, I was completely in love. He stood on my doorstep, uncharacteristically mysterious. "I'm sorry—I just couldn't wait," he said, and reached into his jeans pocket.

I stared as he slowly withdrew something that fit in the palm of his hand. My heart raced. *He's going to propose!* I thought—terrified and elated. Reflexively, I finger-combed my hair and stared ruefully down at my Sunday-night sweats. Dammit! Why wasn't I wearing a cuter outfit? Now I'd have a sweatpants-clad, bra-less, makeup-less, less-than-my-most-attractive-self proposal story to tell everyone.

Then pure panic struck. I was a year out of college. I was too young to settle down. "No! No! I'm not ready!" I said on account of both outfit and age.

"I know, but I have to," he said as he took a deep breath and met my eyes. "Sara, I don't think we should be together anymore."

He opened his hand. There was my key.

I think I stopped breathing. It was my first real love and my first heartbreak. The dark, aching pain caught me unaware; I'd left myself unguarded against this possibility. I had really let someone in, and he had taken a good, long look around and decided this, or rather I, wasn't for him. It was rejection at its deepest, most personal, and intimate level.

I plummeted into the netherworld of post-breakup depression. I lost my notable appetite and withered away to a fraction of a person. The plague of insomnia—ever-faithful ambulance chaser to the scene of a breakup—wasn't far behind.

Robotically, I shifted between home and the office, where I worked as a marketing assistant at a small, crappy brokerage firm that was in the process of being "merged" with a much larger firm. There, I completed each brain-numbing task, attended each brain-numbing meeting, and neither noticed, nor cared about, any part of anything. I was on autopilot, mindlessly drifting through each day.

The fact that it was winter in Boston and the average daily temperature hovered around a biting 20 degrees only made me want to huddle indoors more. The ever-mounting snow drifts, dingy gray from traffic and general city grime, had hardened under additional layers of unyielding ice, thus narrowing the city's sidewalks into one-person lanes on an endless frozen Slip'n Slide. It was my second winter in New England, but without the exhilaration of those first few blissful months of a new relationship, for the first time I really felt the cold.

I basically became a recluse, wrapped up in the cocoon of my favorite fleece blanket and insulated as much from the frigid weather outside as the hollow, frozen ache in my chest. I never wanted to leave my apartment and could barely drag myself to work. To be fair, it wasn't a far leap. My work in the world of financial marketing felt intrinsically meaningless on the best of days.

I'd realized as soon as I started, that neither I, nor the world, nor any of its inhabitants derived any value whatsoever from what I did. This was a sobering and depressing realization. The weight of knowing that this was my life and I was wasting it weighed on me like the Earth on Atlas' shoulders. That I wrestled with these sort of angst-y dilemmas made it clear that I was one of those whale-saving, bad-guy-hunting, human-rights-reporting geeks who actually needed to care about what I did, who needed to believe that what I did helped people in some way. *In any way.*

But I was powerless to do anything about it. I needed a job that would pay the bills and college loans, and finance was the industry that was hiring in Boston after I graduated. So I took the job, shut my mouth, and tried to stop my brain from worrying about it.

This was the beginning of my descent into the trap that is financial services. The gravity of its clutches, it turned out, would far outlast the temporary, but smarting, grief of getting dumped. But I didn't know that then.

Instead, deep in my heartbreak, I found myself sitting at an oversized, scarred, and mangled wooden desk, utterly alone in the middle of a huge empty space outside everyone else's offices, without even a cubicle to provide the illusion of dignity and importance—let alone a shred of privacy, slaving over a weekly internal-only bulletin. I didn't think it could get any worse.

Until it did. The CEO announced that the much larger company with which we were merging was making some "tough calls." The sales guys and their clients would be retained. Pretty much everyone else was let go. I got two weeks of pay and was escorted by security to the door with a box of my personal items.

Stunned and numb, I stood outside the big building, trying to absorb the fact that I was jobless. Naively, I hadn't seen this coming. Layoffs, it seemed, were an awful lot like breakups, which was fitting because dating is awfully similar to working. Sure, it all starts off rosily enough at the first date or interview stage…you shave your legs, wear your best outfit, do your hair and makeup, and sit across from a stranger who you proceed to try to impress with a steady stream of witty banter as you get to know each other. Both parties carefully conceal the downsides they bring to the table. You hide all the difficult, annoying, uncool things about yourself, and the HR rep assures you that being a marketing assistant is totally fun and challenging. Your date, on the other hand, will hide the fact that he's challenging.

You start to date/take the job, and both relationships progress similarly. At first, all parties are on their best behavior. But nobody can stay on best behavior indefinitely. You start to wear your more-comfortable/less-fabulous outfits to work and with your now-boyfriend. You relax about your hair and makeup. Things get comfortable and this seems great because you're in it for the *long haul*.

Or at least I was in it for the long haul. My ex-boyfriend, it seemed, was not. It should've come as no surprise then that I found myself similarly discarded by my employer.

Toting the box of things from my desk, including a framed picture of my ex that I hadn't had the heart to change yet, I plodded slowly home. Walking any faster seemed overwhelming. And thus I was unable to avoid conversing with my gym-rat downstairs neighbor who was universally feared by everyone in the building for being excessively chatty. It was well known that if you went past her unfailingly-open door at anything less than a moderate jog, she'd ensnare you with a verbal barrage about her ever-changing workout obsessions, her 18-year-old cat, or her unerringly strange array of podiatric maladies.

But a moderate jog might as well have been light speed for me. I could barely move at all. And so she caught me, and in the ensuing onslaught which also included details about her incurable toenail fungus, she happened to mention that she'd recently started doing yoga.

From within my desolate gray bleakness, I felt a mild twinge of interest. I'd always wanted to try yoga, without knowing much about it. Connotations of incense, vague spirituality, and unwashed hippie tea drinkers who twisted themselves into pretzels while balancing on one pinky came to mind. Even though I was a well-scrubbed corporate four-cups-a-day coffee drinker, I was intrigued enough to accept her invitation to tag along to her class that night. The fact that I was willing to risk hearing more about her workouts/cat/foot ailments on the commute was indicative of the precise level of my desperation.

The class was in the basement of her gym, in a dark and soon-to-be very sweaty room crowded with yoga mats. There was no incense, but as the class got underway, I might've wished there was.

My neighbor, wearing the world's tiniest shorts and matching bra top, skipped to the front row and beckoned for me to join her. Wearing my baggiest, shabbiest sweats, I shook my head and shuffled to the very back.

I stepped onto the public mat and tried not to think of the stale, vaguely moist, sweat-soaked rubber crawling with God-knows-what microbes. I looked down. My bare feet were a novelty in the middle of the Boston winter. They looked oddly pale, having not seen flip-flops or sun for over four long months. The imprint of my shoes was traced into the tops of my feet where my high heels had cut into them all day, and the red indentations stood in especially stark contrast to the winter-white translucence of my skin, otherwise unmarked except for the purplish veins snaking along their length. I wiggled my toes. They were unpolished. Whoever saw them when they were crammed into work shoes or winter boots? Especially now that I was single, there was no reason to keep up such maintenance.

The thought only made me feel more alone and miserable.

The teacher, a French-Indian woman, had a mesmerizing accent with a particular, melodious way of enunciating each syllable of every word. It created an intoxicating, songlike way of speaking. It seemed so much more authentic to be taking yoga with her than some fake blond with a Boston accent.

She brought her own space heaters and they threw an unrelenting blast of hot air at us. I loved it. I wanted to hurl myself on top of their orange-y glow and start to thaw my sad, frozen bones.

She was short and muscular, with dark skin and a regal carriage, a tiny yoga queen gliding around her hot yoga kingdom. Then, suddenly, she was beside me. Startled, I looked down at her outstretched palm in front of my chin.

"How you gonna breathe with *thees sheet* in your mouth? *Huh*?" she growled.

I'd forgotten that I was chewing gum. I looked for a tissue to place it in. There was none. I gestured and shrugged to explain.

"Geeve it to me, *now*," she commanded, open palm under my chin.

Slightly afraid, I did as I was told. I spit the gum in my new teacher's hand. "And no food for three hours before practice," she added accusingly as though she knew about my last-minute-I-better-eat-*something* spaghetti. I was doubly mortified as she glided to the front and class began.

Around me, everyone stood and began emanating a strange, rhythmic breathing. It sounded hoarse and whispery. The teacher spoke of trying to make this *ujjiy* breath sound like the ocean's waves rushing in to the shore, an inviting image that I had no idea how to execute. I looked right and left, trying to catch an eye, ask for help. Nobody looked back. Feeling foolish and self-conscious, I tried, but it ended up sounding more like strangulation. I tried again, but the back of my throat became dry and my breath caught instead of glided, forcing me into a coughing spasm. *Wow— even breathing is hard in yoga.* I gave up trying to make the proper sound, instead letting my breath fall into a regular deep rhythm. But around me, the *ujjiy* was quietly soothing in its oceanic, cadenced pace.

The poses, flowing from one to the next, felt foreign to my body. The Sanskrit names were foreign to my ears. In fact, everything here felt foreign. But as she pronounced *ev-er-y sin-gle syl-la-ble* with her deep, velvety voice tinged with that musical accent, I felt myself being reeled in.

Little did I know, this was an advanced-level *ashtanga* class and I was hopelessly weak. My arms trembled under my own body weight and my stomach sagged toward the borrowed mat, lacking the core strength to hold myself up as we transitioned from high to low plank—essentially the descent portion of a push-up.

As we moved to the seated portion of class and did the final core work in the primary series, I was unable to sit and hold my legs and torso in a "V" formation for boat pose, *navasana*. My legs shook. The area where my abs should've been shook. Even my arms shook. As the class closed in on 90 minutes, my entire body was quivering from overexertion, but the yogis around me continued callisthenically twisting and contorting themselves into pose after pose.

I transitioned to the final resting pose, *savasana*, with tremendous gratitude that the strenuous portion of class was over and I had made it through. Silently, I celebrated my survival. As I lay quietly on my mat, I thought of my boyfriend—then winced as I mentally corrected myself to think of him as my *ex-boyfriend*—for the first time since the class had begun. Immediately, thoughts of my *ex-job* followed. Burning tears welled up and slid silently down to intermingle with the sweat on my neck.

Still though, as anyone who's been on the receiving end of a breakup, a layoff, or the breakup-layoff double whammy can attest, your ex and your misery are the *only* things you can think of in those first raw weeks. Not thinking of him or it for an hour and a half was the longest and most peaceful respite I'd had from my whirling brain and the aching loneliness since he'd said, "Sara...I don't think..." and my company had shortly followed suit.

I realized with astonishment that I hadn't thought of anything outside of the poses I'd been pitifully attempting during the entire length of this class—a drastic change for my typically racing brain, which vacillated wildly between loving, long-ing thoughts of him, panic about being unemployed, and random tangents every few seconds. *What if I don't find another job? What if I can't pay my student loans? No. Don't think of him...don't think about jobs....God, I miss him. No. Think of this class. Think. Of. This. Class! I should reward myself with mango sorbet. Mmmm...mangos...my Aunt Joan's favorite...did I ever call her back? I wonder how her vacation was....Vacation. If I ever find another job, I should go somewhere. Maybe Greece...white buildings, blue roofs...no, Costa Rica! Exotic frogs! Great beaches! No, Mexico!*

Like most of us, my brain couldn't stay still for more than a few seconds—then it was off to another string of thoughts/worries/to-do lists. Often, I couldn't even retrace my mental steps. How sad is that, really? I mean, *really*?

But because this class had been so physically strenuous and everything so new, it had required all of my concentration to *simply be aware of what was happening at that exact moment* just to attempt to get my weary, untrained body through it. This phenomenon—simply being aware, instead of worrying about events ahead or reliv-ing events behind—was, for me, a novel concept I'd later learn was called "being present."

Physical activity may have been over, but the class was not. The no-nonsense yoga queen gently guided us through a meditation, telling us to visualize ourselves as fish. I fretted briefly over what color fish I should be before settling on a vivid tur-quoise. She guided us to visualize seeing other fish...a striped one...a yellow one...and then to sink to the bottom of the sea and rest. She came around, lifted my head, and with a firm but gentle pull, lengthened my neck. It was the perfect parting gift.

I was so relaxed that I didn't even worry germophobically (as I normally would) about cross-contamination from the other sweaty heads she'd touched. I felt peaceful, like the ocean was cradling me, like the mat, the floor, the yoga itself was holding and supporting me. I never wanted to emerge.

Time passed, but I had no concept of it. An hour? From within the endless space between minutes, there was no telling. At some point, she brought us out of this relaxation and up to sitting. She bowed her head toward the class. Reflexively, I bowed back.

"Wel-come, my new peo-ple, to the yoga practice" she said melodiously, her voice like a gentle island breeze, soothing my battered, bruised heart, even as I wondered why everyone always seemed to call it a "practice," instead of a class or just simply yoga itself. "Go home. Take a *long, hot sho-wer*. Tomorrow *ev-er-y sin-gle mus-cle* in your bo-dy is gonna be sore. But eet's a good sore. See you next week." She smiled, a wide, joyous smile.

The regulars chuckled. I smiled back, totally blissed out, or maybe just punchy from sheer exhaustion.

My neighbor popped up beside me, exuding only slightly less bouncy energy. "Hey! Wanna work out now? You know, weights and cardio?"

Still in my bubble, I shook my head. There was no way I was going to risk losing this yoga bliss even *if* my body had been capable of further activity, which it most certainly was not.

The noise, grime, and jostling of public transportation didn't bother me on the T-ride home, instead it seemed oddly soothing. As instructed, when I got home, I took a "long, hot sho-wer" and crawled into bed, where for the first time since the breakup, I fell into a deep and restful sleep.

The next morning, *ev-er-y sin-gle mus-cle in my bo-dy* was indeed sore. But it was a good sore. I felt accomplished and strong. I'd survived an advanced-level yoga class. I had been initiated into an ancient tradition. And I was already craving another hit of that completely relaxed, physically exhausted peace I'd reveled in at the end of class.

I knew then that I was completely hooked.

Part One:

Corporate Enslavement

Chapter One

Blandular Fever

S *uicide is not an option. The windows in this building don't even open,* I tell myself as I sit in yet another brain-numbing corporate meeting. It's just another day in my brain-numbing, corporate existence.

It's been five years since that first blissful yoga class, and things have improved on the relationship front. After a few more failed attempts, I've finally managed to accidentally meet the double trifecta—tall, dark, and handsome plus respectful, devoted, and kind. But in the career department, I'm still mired in the muck of financial services. This muck has only gotten worse while under the management of a series of stupendously bad bosses. Daily, the urge to stab myself in the head with a letter opener presents itself.

All told, I've learned three things:

1. Neither a broken heart nor a series of crazy bosses and shitty jobs will kill you. They should. But they don't.
2. Sheer determination to gut through a brain-numbing, shitty job can be a seriously powerful thing.
3. While concentrating on gutting through said brain-numbing, shitty job, you can lose years of your life.

In and of itself, a lackluster corporate career might—*might*—be manageable. But in combination with working for my latest bad boss, Vicky, work-life (and given that most of my waking life is spent at work, really just *life*) was quickly reaching an untenable point.

I've only worked at Investorcap for a few months, having changed jobs under the mistaken assumption that it was my prior firm and not the industry that was the problem, but I'd learned in the first few days, with a mixture of fear and wonder, that there is nothing this woman loves more than attention—and nothing she won't do to get it. Vicky wasn't beautiful, but she was unique. In flagrant disregard to unspoken corporate rules (female minority must look as unfeminine as possible!), she wore her dark red hair down past her shoulders. Through unrelentingly regimented eating, Vicky maintained a pin-thin frame. "It helps me get roles," she was often overheard saying. A community theater fanatic, she proudly displayed photos of herself in various theatrical performances all over her office. She'd seemed artsy and cool in the sea of corporate sameness I'd been swimming in for years. Initially, I had admired her.

But that quickly gave way to a feeling of dread as it became clear that her professional life was yet another stage on which Vicky wanted to star as the diva. Clues started accumulating pretty early on that maybe things weren't going to be as good as I'd hoped—snarky comments about what I ate: ("Wow. You're eating *again*?! Aren't you adorable!" "You're ordering dessert? How *robust* of you. I'm just so full from my salad...") and how I dressed: ("Those are *interesting* shoes. They look like knock-offs of a pair of Manolos I had six seasons ago..."). I let them roll off; I'd come to expect that from corporate females.

But other alarming behaviors were harder to dismiss. In a recent red-flag escapade, she'd performed miniskirted, crotch-flashing, chorus-line kicks as a "warm-up exercise" on the podium at a conference, later subjecting fellow conference attendees to her throaty rendition of old show tunes on an hour-long shuttle bus ride. To be clear, this was not an understated performance—Vicky's shuttle bus soundtrack was best likened to that of a drag queen impersonating Judy Garland as she belted out the grand finale of, "Ollllllld Maaaaaaaaan Riiiiiiiverrrrrrr." These sorts of antics irrefutably depicted her predilection for the spotlight. She was a caricature whose behavior was so ludicrous she didn't seem real. But she was real...and, even more disturbing, she was my boss.

Valiantly trying not to worry about this sur-reality or the sinking feeling that I should've stayed in the last frying pan, I attempt to tune in to the meeting…this brutally inane, wretchedly boring meeting.

"Guys…and, uh, ladies," Charles, the head of the entire sales and marketing department, aka the "big boss," Vicky's boss, clears his throat and nods his bald head at Vicky and me to smooth over his grudging acknowledgment that there are, in fact, two females present. "Let's talk NYC. Guys, we gotta bring the A-game. We've got the portfolio guys down there today, sales guys there Friday, and marketing goes down tomorrow. You're all set, right, Vicky?" And with that, the all-male rhetoric comes to a screeching halt.

Wearing a skin-tight custom-made button down, Vicky arches her back to best advantage and peers over her glasses. "Already on it," she purrs.

Charles seems unswayed by the display. "Sara going with you?"

My head snaps up almost as fast as Vicky's face hardens. "Oh, I don't think that's nec—"

"Gotta get her out in the field, Vick," Charles snaps. "Okay….Walshy, you're up, buddy!" He claps Walshy on the back affectionately—a gesture that's never afforded to Vicky or me. Women are also left out of the buddy-buddy practice of being referred to by last name or variations thereof. The incongruous truth was that in spite of well-known scandalous stripper escapades and rampant philandering on the road, the male majority lives in fear of a career-ending harassment claim within the office. They're excruciatingly careful how they speak to the token corporate females. Affectionate claps are out of the question.

As Walshy makes his way to the whiteboard, I stare carefully down at my notepad. Vicky's obvious reluctance to take me only reaffirms my conclusion that she isn't going to be a good mentor. Which is super disappointing since I'd taken this job precisely because she had seemed to be exactly what I was looking for. At 40, she was already tremendously successful: the head of marketing and a Senior Vice President. (It's standard in the corporate world to capitalize titles even though they are not proper nouns in an attempt, I can only imagine, to make oneself Feel More Important.)

Vicky was only one level away from Executive Vice President, a level of corporate enlightenment that bordered on urban legend among females as I'd never actually met one and nobody I knew had either. The first time I met her, Vicky had let it be known she intended to achieve EVP status. As a Director, two levels below her, my goal was to reach VP. I'd hoped she could show me how. Her initial praise had seemed so promising.

"You're Italian?" she'd murmured approvingly during my interview a few months back, eyeing my last name. "Italians are the most elegant and sophisticated people on Earth. Nobody knows food and wine like the Italians."

Even while hoping that this made it more likely I'd get the job, I'd stifled my instinct to be flattered, noting that her surname was Italian as well. It had seemed safest to say nothing, and especially nothing about those *other* Europeans who've been known to dabble in food and wine.

"I myself am actually half Italian," she'd continued, either reading my mind or forgetting I was there. "Father Italian, mother Icelandic. Thank God. The Icelandic side gives me a cooler head and temper. And this red hair. Men *love* red hair." Interestingly, her allegedly Icelandic-derived red hair had jet-black roots.

I should've known when Vicky offered me the job over lunch at the Ritz, during which she had seemed far more interested in her side salad and hefty glass of wine than in me, that she was not interested in elevating my career. I was too thrilled—to be presented with a job offer! at the Ritz!—to notice. I'd accepted immediately.

Coming up on nearly a decade in financial services, I've sat in my fair share of pointless meetings and worked for my fair share of bad female bosses. But although the particulars of the building, company, boss, or conference room may have changed, the substance of life within work has stayed constant. As usual, I'm either the only woman or, occasionally, one of two women in the room. All the men in the meeting—a sliver but accurately representative of all the men I've ever worked

14

with—look the same: middle-aged white guys in custom-tailored suits with thinning hair and expanding guts. They're slight variations of one another, all sporting the same wildly overpriced silk ties imprinted with sailboats, lobsters, or golf themes, and the same shirts varying only in the width of the pinstripe and whether the cuffs are French or buttons. All of them tolerate, with varying degrees, our female presence.

I zone in and out as Walshy, oozing intense, highly caffeinated excitement, goes for the gold in trying to cram as many industry buzz words into his time on the floor as possible. "Alright guys, let's step up to the plate and whiteboard it. The pipeline's looking strong; performance is up. All wins, guys, all wins. There's no "I" in team, am I right guys? Am I right? Now here's where the rubber meets the road....We need to strategize, synergize, get our ducks in a row, and add value on an apples-to-apples basis. So let's keep it going and make an extra effort for our new client in New York! Joe—nice work reeling that one in, buddy. Air fist bump! *Blowing* it up! Yeah! I like that. Now let's really grab 'em by the balls, bring 'em to their knees, show those guys who their daddy is. Then go for the low-hanging fruit...."

I try not to visibly drool on myself.

For all I know, this guy could be talking about synergizing the swinging of his right and left balls, his own variation of "low-hanging fruit." That, at least, would be more interesting.

If I feel a little guilty for mentally straying from the minutiae of the performance data at hand, I comfort myself by remembering that zoning out is actually a survival tactic and a protection mechanism for the safety and well-being of my fellow employees. If I actually tuned in, if I fully subjected myself to this drivel, day in and day out, year after year, I could go postal. No, I *would*, most certainly, go postal. As in, have a total flipping meltdown. Paint myself a warrior face with Wite-Out and embark on a Rambo-like, chest-pounding, pen- and legal-pad hurling, dry-erase-marker-snorting, feet-stomping, hair-ripping rampage where I'd likely end up splattered on the inside of the conference room window like a bug on a windshield, unceremoniously halted in the middle of a desperate attempt to get the hell out of here.

In my haste, I'd almost certainly neglect to note that the window isn't a designated emergency exit, which the Operating Committee to Recognize and Prepare for Possible Emergencies/Disasters (or, as I liked to think of them, O-CRAPPED) had educated us on during the O-CRAPPED conference. I probably missed that little detail about the window/non-exit, having been much too busy coming up with the O-CRAPPED acronym.

The sales guy to my right, who refers to himself as "The Meat," stands up for the classic "male adjust"—his signature move during meetings—then starts speaking without waiting to be acknowledged. "Walshy, buddy, listen. Walshy, if I may…this top-down revenue model reminds me of a case study I led at HBS, uh, that'd be Harvard Business School for all you non-alums," he punctuates this with a condescending chuckle. This is a necessary corporate moment—it isn't officially a meeting until The Meat brings up his alma mater. "And I have some thoughts I'd like to share with the group."

My mind wanders again as The Meat drones on. My non-reaction to my colleague actually calling himself "The Meat" indicates I've worked in finance for far too long. As I rotate my ankle in circles and then figure eights, I wonder, not the first time, *What am I doing here?*

Wait. Rewind the tape. *Where* am *I?*

An overwhelming feeling of not belonging engulfs me. Even my gray pinstripe suit and gorgeous patent leather wedge heels—a celebratory purchase after my last promotion—feel restrictive. They're a wool and leather form of shackles.

In spite of this, I smile affectionately at the shiny, black-patent-leather, five-inch-wedge heels gleaming up at me. These shoes are to me what phone booths are to Clark Kent. I become a different person in them. Sure, like most heels, I can't walk any distance in them, and they contract my Achilles tendon while jacking my feet up at an unnatural angle like a Barbie foot. And, okay fine, I'm sure they probably also compress my lower back. *But* I always get at least one compliment every time I wear them, and I feel fabulous and stylish in them.

Walsh manages to wrest the meeting back from The Meat. Though they may be buddies, they're still competitors. Drunk on the success of recommandeering the spotlight, he celebrates by blathering relentlessly on about sales projections. I take advantage of the conference room's view, gazing out at Boston Harbor.

The problem with my job, public relations, is that I never actually *create* anything. Therefore, I never actually have any concrete results to show for myself at the end of the day. What I do is very abstract. Like most middle managers, I attend meetings. I liaise, I manage, I oversee, I organize, I supervise, I synergize. But you can't feel, see, or touch that. I can't step back at the end of the day, week, year, or decade and say, "Look, here's what I've accomplished!" in the same way that you can step back after a day of planting or building, and actually *see* what you've accomplished.

When you get down to brass tacks, what I do is also pretty meaningless...like this meeting. And if it doesn't wrap up soon I'm going to have to consider a more desperate means of escape. I glance longingly toward the window, but think better of it.

Ugh, I hate this boring, endless meeting. Ugh, I hate financial services.

And here's another reason why: financial services has been built into the monstrosity that it is based entirely on making things more enormous and complicated than the industry or its products ever actually needed to be. Yes, there is *some* need for financial services in its more basic form, as people (myself very much included) need help with financial planning. But there should not be the number of advisers or products that currently exist. Most of them are crowding the market with their presence and they know damn well that what they have to offer is subpar.

Investorcap—or as I like to think of it, Invest-o-crap—is both a prime example and a microcosm of the broader financial services industry, the majority of which is run by individuals who vary between corrupt and just plain inept. Yet, like the majority of the industry, we continue to elbow our way into the frenzy. The reason for this is simple. Despite the "we care about our customer" facade, all these companies really want to do is make money. If they really cared about the customer, the sales guys would have to say, "Listen, despite the fact that I want your business, I'm ethically obligated to tell you the best product in its class is actually available through our competitor."

But who'd ever say that? It's like hoping a used car dealer will tell you that the best bang for your buck is actually available from their competitor across the street.

So instead, in true corporate style, these companies take stock of their cruddy products and initiate multi-million-dollar advertising campaigns to figure out ways to entice the public into buying said cruddy products. I know this because I'm on the advertising committee that designs those campaigns. And while it's interesting and exciting to create commercials that millions of people see on national television, it leaves me feeling a bit more hollow to know that I'm part of perpetuating this lie.

And so, as I sit here in this stupor-inducing sales and marketing synergization meeting, hearing about infinitesimal, two-bps ("bps" standing for basis points, each of which equals one one-hundredth of a percent, an amount otherwise too small to measure) changes in fund performance, I ponder the larger issue. And that is that I can't feel good about what I do or who I work with.

The problem is that most people don't go into financial services for a sheer love of it the way, say, some people join the Peace Corps or want to save the whales. Financial services attracts people who love money and want to get rich. Too often, they are sleazy, paunchy sales guys who turn over receipts to their young, usually female, assistants to transform into expense reports for the steaks they gluttonously feast on, the booze they swill, the strippers they hire, the private dances they get, and maybe even the hookers they later have back to their rooms—all in the name of entertaining the client of course. And this isn't just one rogue dude. No, this is a shockingly large portion of the male-dominated financial services industry.

Of course, not every guy is like this. There are probably some wonderful guys who are devoted to their families and who actually believe in what they do. (This boggles my mind, but is most assuredly true.) But unfortunately, they're too hard to find because when what you do is solely devoted to the altar of monetary gain, then why not try to milk the system? It's not like you're taking money away from orphans, right?

18

Maybe. But frankly, there are only so many years that a person can work in this environment, surrounded by and immersed in it each day for far more hours than one is with one's family or friends, before, at some point, one's soul starts to feel sullied…and then slowly begins to erode.

Or at least that's how *this* person felt. Maybe others can thrive—in fact, I'm utterly sure they can because they *do*. And that is who comprises the senior sales and management teams at major companies like this one.

And if they can live with themselves, fine. However, the longer I work in this industry, the clearer it's becoming that I can't trudge along like this for three more decades. I already volunteer, raising money to build schools in Africa and tutoring an underprivileged child in Boston, but maybe I need to actually work for a do-good organization. Unfortunately, the inherent pay cut falls somewhere between merely unappealing and completely terrifying. Made even more so by the fact that I'm entirely out on my own—my mother died from cancer and I have no relationship with my father.

Not having a parental safety net, whether the webbing is financial, emotional, or some interwoven combination, steers not only the course of anyone's life but also each of the many choices of which it's comprised. Knowing there wasn't a safety net under my world, and keenly feeling the absence of its protection, influenced every decision. I'd grown up dirt poor, worked my way through college, and was, for the first time in my life, enjoying the freedom of self-reliance and whatever modicum of financial security I could scrape together. The idea of relinquishing any degree of that sense of safety was too scary to fully consider.

Turning my mind away from these gloomy reflections, I focus instead on thoughts of attending a yoga class after work. In the years since my initiation, yoga had served in equal measure as both a sanctuary and a savior. It was a place where I could burn off the ick of the day and emerge rejuvenated…just in time to run straight back into the burning barn that was my career. Just as any body rearranges itself around its limitations—adjusting to hunching, limping, or chronic pain until it becomes such an innate part of yourself that you don't remember a time when it wasn't there, I'd folded myself around chronic career misery and learned to lean on yoga like a crutch. This was far easier than investing the inestimable work and time to figure out what I really wanted—and could realistically do—with my life.

I'm picturing sweeping my arms up for the first sun salutation when Charles unexpectedly asks me to report on the public relations effort of which I am the Director. Panic washes over me and settles in my lower belly. It's in knots. Charles has never asked me to report to the group. Public relations is only a priority when something horrible happens. When a CEO is fired, fund managers stage a walkout, or performance tanks, I suddenly become visible. When the crisis passes, I fade back into obscurity. Happily.

I swallow nervously. Being caught off guard leads me to the ultimate corporate blunder: honesty. "Things are pretty tough right now. One of our affiliates may be the subject of an undercover media investigation about packaging and selling subprime mortgages. Due to our relationship, naturally this could lead to bad press for us as well. There's nothing we can really do to control the story as it is *undercover* and I don't know when—or even if—it will break."

Charles glares at me, and my heart drops. Then he ignores completely, and somehow, that's even scarier. He's pissed—*really* pissed, and I'm in trouble—*serious* trouble. I suddenly remember that the importance of honesty, much like teamwork, is a myth in the modern workplace.

Unfortunately, I'm compulsively honest. Which basically mean I'm screwed. The knots in my stomach tighten. I feel sick over my impending confrontation and reprimand. There is nothing worse than waiting for the ax to fall.

Chapter Two
Female Troubles

After the meeting, I wander slowly back to my office and wait nervously for Betsy to call. Betsy, a slender brunette who worked as an admin for the FBI before somehow ending up as the executive assistant for both Vicky and Charles, is one of the two people I most adore at this job. She made the top two when she sat down next to me in one of the first meetings I'd been in and muttered, "Thank God I wore polyester today, now I can strap a feedbag on. Call maintenance if you need help rolling my bloated remains back to my cube." She'd followed this up with an adorably hearty, somewhat diabolical laugh.

I glance up, inadvertently looking across the hall and straight at The Meat, who's reclining in his $1,800 chair, with his Dockers-clad legs up on the desk and his hands behind his head. He wiggles his eyebrows and winks at me. The Meat has a window office and a panoramic view of the harbor. I have an internal office, which was a former filing cabinet room, and a view of...The Meat, which I'm free to enjoy anytime since all offices have glass walls at Investorcap. Our glass walls are a symbol of openness and transparency, the senior management always brags to prospective clients, which is bitterly ironic in that the financial industry sorely lacks both qualities.

A moment later my phone lights up with Betsy's extension. "Sara, he'd like to see you," she says in the strained, ultraprofessional tone that indicates that he's (a) staring directly at her and (b) it is, in fact, really bad. I take a deep breath and head over.

In the 20 seconds it takes me to walk down the hall, Charles is already on another call. I stand nervously outside his office. "Maternity leave is a goddamn joke!" he protests vehemently. "Yeah, my ass—it's a damn paid vacation is what it is...hell no! I wouldn't give it if the damn lawyers weren't all over me with that goddamn Family Leave Act shit...." Slouching lower in his chair as the shoeshine guy kneeling at his feet continues polishing his left loafer, Charles catches a glimpse of me. Deliberately, he looks away again, leaving me marooned until he wraps up his conversation.

"Charles?" I ask brightly when he's finally hung up and the shoeshiner has scurried on to the sales guys. Although I guess I too could hire him, for some reason, only the men in our office do. This is fine by me. I prefer to drop my shoes off to the cobbler instead of having someone kneeling at my feet.

"Close the door," he says tightly. Decades of disapproving have resulted in the loose skin of his cheeks sagging down to his jowls, giving him a disapproving hangdog expression. If everyone has an animal persona, Charles's would be an old bloodhound—from the jowls to his gloomy air.

He does not invite me to sit down. So I stand—hovering awkwardly—while he sits behind his desk and chews me out.

The fact that he never actually raises his voice—the fact that he issues one long diatribe of icy wrath—actually makes it worse. "Our department doesn't want to hear the 'truth,'" he spits out the word disdainfully. "We want to be pumped up with good news. And if there's no good news," he continues tightly, "then spin the news we have, goddammit. Don't you know how to do that? Isn't that what we're *paying* you for? Maybe this company has mistaken you for an experienced professional. *Maybe* I've stuck my neck out for you *time and again* for nothing."

The implication that he'd ever stuck his neck out for me at all shocks me. I swallow. I really want to cry, but I swallow instead. "I thought I should tell the truth. Of course I'm prepared to spin the news for the press and the public, but I thought internal people needed the facts. I didn't want to withhold information from people senior to me....I thought I was doing the right thing."

Apparently, I'm wrong. "We want happy! We want peppy!" He gestures with a sort of pom-pom shaking with his hands, then impales me with his stare. "We want to feel great after we hear from our PR girl—*great* about where we work, great about what we do!" He looks at the floor, his voice is dark and low. "Today was an embarrassment. An embarrassment to yourself. And an embarrassment to me. Don't ever, *ever* let that happen again."

As upset as I am by this whole episode, I'm most frustrated with myself. *Ugh.* *"PR girl." When will I ever get it?* I've been at this game too long—almost a decade now—to allow myself to be tripped by such rookie mistakes. If I was on top of my game or had had time to prepare, I would've remembered that you never give them what they *ask for*—you give them what they actually *want*.

So I take the reprimand like a man. No tears and no slinking out. I lift my head and stare him in the eye. If I've learned one thing it's that men don't really want women in the workplace—at least not in this industry, at least not in the workplaces I know. And if a woman *must* be there, then please, don't act like a woman—like Vicky does for instance, and which everyone (especially other women) hates her for doing.

I ignore all the inquiring glances from my colleagues as I walk past their offices. In a department where emails go around about Charles's mood "stormy today—beware" or "sunny and clear today—quick! Ask for what you need!" it's not small news when he pulls someone in and closes the door. They're dying to know what went down and my tearstained or smiling face will yield valuable clues.

The gossipy nature of this office is even more irritating when I'm the subject of its inquiry. Carefully, I keep my face impassive, revealing nothing. I shut my door and refresh my email, focusing intently on the screen. I calculate exactly how many minutes until I can go out into the bitter cold night and make my way to yoga. My yoga craving is strong—matched only by my desire to get out of this place.

Abruptly, there's a sharp rap on my door and before I can look up or signal entry, Vicky barges in.

She skips any pleasantries. "Clear your calendar for New York. We might as well throw in a visit with that PR firm you hired too." The derisiveness in her voice when she refers to "that PR firm *you* hired," makes it clear—in case her direct comments to the same effect hadn't already—that she thinks my choice of firm was a huge mistake.

For reasons I don't understand, she radiates hostility. "We'll leave for the airport tomorrow at three." With a final withering glare, she pivots on one stiletto and slams the door behind her.

Ugh. I hate my boss. I hate my job. I hate financial services.

Chapter Three
A Day in the Life of a Worker Bee

We meet our new PR agency president and account exec for dinner at an *über-chic* Manhattan restaurant. The kind with low lights and sparse, modern furnishings that exude an indefinable air of fabulousness. As the Director of Public Relations at Investorcap, a major industry player with billions under management, I'd been brought on board to expand the company's presence in the media. In order to launch this new initiative, my first order of business had been to hire a firm to assist me. Now it was time for that firm to reassure me (and my disapproving boss) that I'd made the right decision, and that their $20,000 a month retainer was money well spent.

Conversation consists of the usual corporate tail-fanning of who you know and where you've worked. Shortly after downing a final cappuccino, the president of the agency dashes off to catch the train back to New Jersey and his family, leaving me alone with Vicky and Samantha, our account exec, who'd worked her way through college modeling in Milan. With a thick fall of platinum blond hair, the largest, bluest eyes I've ever seen, and an immaculately toned 5'11" body, Samantha had every straight male in the vicinity craning to check her out.

I'd liked Samantha immediately because she'd identified herself as a fellow yoga doer and complimented me on my shoes. This was the jackpot of future friendship potential.

Vicky, however, didn't care for the competition. She'd narrowed her eyes suspiciously and swept the room with a glance to assess if attention was being diverted to Samantha. It wasn't even a close call. Next to Samantha, Vicky looked painfully emaciated and old. Her designer clothes hung limply off her bony frame and deep lines crept through her expensive makeup.

"Get a load of that schnozz," Vicky mutters under her breath after Samantha excuses herself to say hello to the CEO of a company even larger than ours. "I don't see how she could've modeled with a nose like that."

"I didn't notice," I lie, just to move on. But I *had* noticed and Samantha's nose was model-perfect.

"You didn't?! How could you have missed it? That thing's *huge*! And her pants are *way* too tight. See how they hug her butt like that? *See*?" She puts her wineglass down long enough to make a much-too-graphic cupping gesture, then promptly snatches it back up again and takes a hefty swig of her pinot noir. "Those pants are *very* unprofessional." I briefly wonder if these comments are professional and why Vicky's looking at Samantha's butt and the size of her nose anyway. I also had to wonder if she was this critical of me when I wasn't there. Self-consciously, I run a fingertip down the bridge of my own sizable schnozz.

"So…what's the presentation on tomorrow?" I ask in a desperate effort to get on professional footing.

"Don't worry about that," she snaps, narrowing her eyes. "You're just there to *observe*." She draws out the last word for extra emphasis—as people sometimes do when speaking to those who don't speak their language or who they perceive to be very stupid. As a native English speaker, I have no choice but to put myself in the latter category.

As Samantha returns, Vicky coos, "Sam! Darling! I've ordered another bottle of wine. Now sit down here and tell me every little thing about the dating scene in Manhattan." She pats the chair next to her with a little too much enthusiasm.

I shudder, but Samantha takes it in stride. "Actually, I'm dating a CEO. He has an up-and-coming hedge fund company. I'm pretty excited—I think this could be it."

Vicky's eyes narrow as they swing over to me. "And you?"

I swallow and admit I've been dating a lawyer named Walter Nunnally, whom I call "Nunnally" because I've never really liked the name Walter.

"Tell us about him," Vicky commands, clearly unhappy to be the only one still on the "dating scene."

I ignore my better judgment that personal details shouldn't be shared with a boss and blush, as much from the pleasure of thinking of him as from the vulnerability of talking about our relationship. "Well, he's just wonderful!" I begin. "He's kind and caring and…I guess the best way to describe him is that I once learned in a management workshop that humans, at their most basic level, seek to understand and be understood, and he makes me feel like that—truly known and understood. I don't know—I'm gushing!" I gush, usually the opposite of the kind of girl who gushes.

Vicky narrows her eyes and gazes at me coolly. "I'm psychic," she says unexpectedly. "It runs in my family. I get these feelings. And I'm telling you, *this*." She makes a squiggly motion with her wineglass at me. "*This* won't last." She turns to Samantha. "Sara'll dump this guy and break his heart within six months."

I stare at her. I try not to gape hostilely and probably fail. This was my new *boss*. I couldn't very well tell her to go piss up a rain pipe, but backing down felt like a betrayal to Nunnally. For half a second I wonder if maybe she really is psychic, which is devastating to consider, but stranger things have happened.

"I guess we'll have to wait and see," I finally manage, digging deep for diplomacy. Conversation moves on, but I'm engulfed by an ominous feeling. There is something very wrong with Vicky. I didn't have to be psychic to pick up on that.

Authoritatively, Vicky raises her arm, signaling the waiter for yet another bottle of wine. I, who usually chooses wines by scanning down the right-hand price column, notice Vicky's a left-hand name column orderer, with extremely expensive taste to boot.

Needing a moment from the vortex of this conversation, I excuse myself to the ladies room. In the comforting dim solitude, I smooth on lipstick, layer it with gloss, and straighten my hair. The familiarity of these mundane actions is comforting, confidence-boosting. Stalling for time, I check my suit from all angles in the mirror. To my surprise, I look like a real businesswoman—a real businesswoman out at a real business dinner at a chic restaurant in Manhattan. I actually look the part.

So how come I don't *feel* the part? How come I feel like nothing more than an impostor? Although I try to ignore it, this same sense of not belonging haunts me every single day as I walk through the revolving door into the hushed, marble lobby of my skyscraper office building, ascend the elevator a dizzying 40 floors, and stride into my office where I attempt to pull off the charade that I actually know what I'm doing for one more day.

It boggles my mind, but appears to be true: this 750-billion-dollar company actually trusts me, at the age of 28, to build a PR program for them from the ground up, trusts my judgment that this is the right outside firm to support me in doing so, trusts my decision to hire them, is willing to foot the hundreds of thousands of dollars that the program will cost per year, and actually pays me a very good salary to orchestrate it all. They trust me to do that because I convinced them that I can.

And the funny thing is that I actually *am* doing it. Quite successfully, in fact. So why do I feel like a fake? Why do I feel like I'm getting away with this farce by the skin of my teeth and that it's only a matter of time before they catch me? Am I *actually* managing to pull off this charade? *Really*?

The fact that I really *am* only fills me with anxiety and insecurity.

That I'm good at my job somehow doesn't change my deep-down certainty that I don't belong here. I'm in the wrong place. The wrong company. The wrong industry. I lean against the sink and try valiantly to ignore the fact that this is categorically not what I want to do with my life, or what I feel in my bones that I'm *meant* to do with my life.

"Get it together," I warn my reflection sternly. Where I should be and what I should be doing are unknowable. And there's no time for dillydallying in the realm of what-ifs. This is my career and I should be happy to have it.

Trying to shake off the weight of these thoughts, I reluctantly weave my way back to the table. My career may be the overarching issue, but the immediate problem remains: Vicky.

The kitchen closes and our server, looking relieved, transitions us to the bar area. For the next few hours, Vicky babbles about her acting lessons, her "Find Your Voice, Find Yourself" singing bike tour of Ireland, her passion for growing bonsais, the implosion of her latest relationship, the landscaping of her Maine summer home, her search for a larger downtown condo, and her intention to write a best-selling book about growing bonsais. She had two frontrunners for the title: *Thoughts from a Tiny Tree, Thoughts from Me* and *Lessons Learned from Growing a Tiny Bush: The Importance of Pruning, Maintenance, and Life.* "I'll be on TV soon. You'll see me. Oh, yes. You! Will! See! Me!" She pounds a fist on the table for punctuation.

Quickly, I reach to steady a teetering wineglass.

She rounds on me spastically. "You're not drinking enough," she slurs, leaning in crookedly and leering directly into my eyes.

"I am!" I assure her, trying to disguise my sobriety. A wise employee knows never to be drunker than her boss. In this case, there's no danger of that. I'm stone-cold sober; Vicky is plastered.

Our new server appears with a single martini balanced on a tray. "For the beautiful young lady, compliments of the gentleman at the bar," he says with a French accent and a slight bow to Samantha.

Vicky reaches across the table and snatches it. "Isn't that nice! I'm flattered!" she coos, with a fluttery wave of thanks toward the bar.

The server clears his throat awkwardly. "Actually, *madam*, it was for this young—"

"It's fine," Samantha cuts in quickly. "Tell him Vicky says *thank you.*" Her pointed gaze tells the waiter even more than her firm tone.

The server nods reluctantly and hurries away.

"So...where are you guys staying?" Samantha asks, presumably to buffer an increasingly awkward moment.

Noticeably pleased with this topic, Vicky rears back into her seat, trilling a laugh. "Oh, I only ever stay at the Ritz or the Four Seasons." She looks satisfied, adding confidentially, "I tell the company I don't feel 'safe' anywhere else. And since I'm the only woman in senior management..." her voice trails off and she shrugs carelessly. *I get what I want*, hangs, implied, in the air. And she's right. It could be a career-ending move ("CEM" in corporate vernacular) if male management crossed the token female executive on something that smacked of gender bias—especially if the token female executive was one as demonstrably unstable as Vicky.

The bad feeling in the pit of my stomach grows. *This woman is dangerous*, I think in a moment of insight that only comes when one is confronted with complete, unfettered insanity. *And it's only a matter of time until she turns on me.* Then, it will boil down to a matter of survival. It will be her or it will be me.

Like the distant rumble of thunder heralds an incoming storm, a battle is brewing. Someone will emerge the victor and someone will limp away defeated. She has every advantage: Seniority. Title. Connections. Success. There's also something cold, menacing, and devious about her. As she'd just implied, she gets what she wants.

I'm her subordinate. I'm new. I'm vulnerable. The only thing I have on my side is truth. And from what I know of the corporate world, that usually doesn't amount to much. I swallow hard.

Maybe I'm overreacting. *Rein it in, DiVello.* I try to shake off the sense of foreboding.

At two am, Vicky informs us it's time to leave and swirls her signature at the bottom of the $3,000 tab. Three thousand dollars for dinner for four people—one of whom had dashed out early. Clearly, as she'd inferred, Vicky gets what she wants. *At any cost.*

She tries to rise, but sways drunkenly and quickly sits back down, too unsteady to stand on her own. Mortified in front of Samantha, the waiter, and the still well-populated bar, I half-carry her outside. Samantha, looking something between embarrassed and concerned, hails a cab, and I maneuver Vicky into it despite her alcohol-induced floppiness.

We arrive at the Four Seasons and I guide her to her door. "I'ffff gotit!" she half-snaps, half-slurs, stabbing futilely at the lock with her key card. "Lobby. Eight am," she barks over her shoulder as she finally manages to open the door and stumble inside.

Worried to my bones about her behavior, I head to my own room.

At 8:00 am, I'm dressed and waiting in the lobby. Vicky, however, is nowhere to be seen.

Nervously, I look around for her. If I am in the wrong place, I will suffer the consequences. If I am in the right place but not where she wants me to be, I will still suffer the consequences. Getting frantic, I ask the concierge for messages. I look in the restaurant. Anxiety coursing through me, I check my Blackberry compulsively. Has she changed the time? The location?

At 8:15, I email to ask. At 8:30, I call her room, desperate.

"I'm *on* my *way!*" Click. Dial tone.

Finally, wearing huge, designer sunglasses that take up most of her bony face, she appears and sweeps past me brusquely. "I have the spins. I need to stop for coffee," she announces. Her hands are visibly shaking.

I glance nervously at my watch. We're already late, but I do not dare to argue.

At the coffee shop, she gulps a double espresso, then turns to me. "You're really fine?" she asks, her tone somewhere between doubt and accusation. "I think I'm going to be sick."

I nod, afraid this will only make her madder.

By the time we finally arrive, the all-male room is seated and waiting, the air thick with indignation: *How the hell are these two bimbos late? Don't they know who we are?*

Deliberately—or perhaps woefully—unaware, Vicky issues breezy, insincere apologies alongside double kisses as she slaps her laptop onto the podium and we all wait for it to boot up. In real time, a few moments pass; in feel-real time, a few millenniums pass. Vicky makes her way to the front and clears her throat. Her skin looks pale and waxy. She brushes back her hair, as usual, it's defiantly down and unbound. My own hair is pulled up in a chignon so tight as to induce a headache.

As soon as her PowerPoint presentation flashes onto the screen, Vicky clears her throat again and begins. "Our marketing strategy is based on a four-prong ap-

proach consisting of a $10,000,000 ad campaign, a new public relations initiative—"
She stops abruptly and swallows hard. Her brow is sweaty. "Please excuse me," she
says, hurrying from the room.

The men look around, startled and confused. There is a general rumble of murmurs as to what the hell is going on. I freeze, wondering the same thing. My heart is
pounding. I watch the second hand of the wall clock slog forward as though it's one
of those strong man contestants towing a jet. Five endless minutes later, Vicky returns, muttering, "Such a silly misunderstanding. Let's continue."

Some measure of relief mixes with the anxiety coursing through me. Unfortunately, she only gets to the third page before she claps a hand over her mouth and
runs from the room. "Take over!" she chokes out as she speeds by.

OH MY GOD!

The all-male audience turns to watch her abrupt, scandalous exit. Then eyes
swing to me. I freeze, immobilized. Anxiety skyrockets into pure, blazing panic. My
heart is going too fast. I hear each staccato beat pounding in my ears. It hurts. The
men stare at me and they slide and blur together. There's not enough air. I try to
swallow. The men are still staring. It's too hot in here. I'm teetering on the edge of
passing out or pulling myself back. I have to do this. I dig down, deep into my guts
and grab onto something. This moment. Consciousness. I hold tight. Claw back with
everything I've got.

A long moment passes. Then I'm back, safely away from the edge. I stand. As
Vicky had said, I was here only to *observe*. She hadn't shared anything about the
presentation. I haven't seen the slides. I don't even know the topic. Blushing hotly, I
totter to the front. "Uh…h-hello," I stutter nervously. I look down at the pages, as
much a stranger to their contents as the audience is. "Uh…let's flip to the next page
and see what we have."

Reaching elbow deep into the ass of corporate BS, I somehow bumble haphaz-
ardly through the rest of the 40-odd pages, wrap up the meeting, shake hands with
everyone, and wait nervously for Vicky in reception. She's nowhere to be seen. Giv-

en her unappreciative reaction at the hotel, I don't want to risk calling her again. I check the ladies room in the reception area. No Vicky.

So, I wait. And wait. And…wait. Finally, I make what I hope seems to be a casual loop around the office. On some level, because I want everything to be okay, I hope to find her blithely issuing more double kisses or perched in her short skirt on the edge of a C-level exec's desk laughing off this morning's "misunderstanding." But I find nothing of the kind. The only other possible explanation is that she ditched me and flew back to Boston, which certainly seemed possible given the mind-bending shenanigans of the trip so far.

"Are there any other bathrooms on this floor?" I finally ask the receptionist doubtfully.

"There's another set of restrooms, but they haven't been updated yet," she says. "We're in the middle of major renovations." There's no sign of construction, but I take her word for it.

I walk down two hallways of offices to find said older bathrooms. I peek in nervously. And there she is: sprawled like a ragdoll on the tile floor in the handi-capped stall. The acrid smell of alcohol and vomit assaults my nose, mixing with the scent of industrial cleaners that seem to be an integral fixture of any public restroom.

"Vicky? Are you okay?" I ask hesitantly.

She moans an unintelligible response.

"Can I…um…do anything?"

She moans again, pointing vaguely toward the paper towel dispenser.

I kneel on the cold tile floor and dab her forehead with the requested paper towels. Silently, she conveys that she'll allow me the honor of doing this, closing her eyes with a smug little grin.

"Do you want to go to a doctor?" I ask, sitting back on my heels.

"No…no. You'll just take care of me."

Panic spikes. "I'm not really qualified…you seem really sick. I think we should go to the ER?" I hate that it sounds like a question. Hate that I'm too afraid to put her crazy drunk ass in a cab and head for the nearest hospital in spite of her protests.

She shakes her head. "No! No hospital. I'm fine!" Pale, sweaty, and reeking of vomit, she doesn't *look* fine.

I dab her forehead and comb the matted hair off her face. A few minutes later, she passes out. I sit back against the wall and, like a new mother, watch her breathe, terrified she'll suddenly stop. The seconds slip slowly into minutes, then an hour. Still passed out, she moans, knitting her brows together. *What if she's not just drunk? What if she dies? What the hell will I do if she dies?*

I sneak out to the lobby to call Nunnally at his office. Nunnally always seems to know what to do, no matter how bizarre or extreme the situation. Halfway through moving us into our apartment, one of our movers had started feeling dizzy. Nunnally had taken his pulse, detected an irregular heartbeat, and promptly driven the mover to the nearest emergency room, where he was immediately admitted for a serious arrhythmia. If Nunnally could stay calm through that, a drunk boss shouldn't even register on the Richter scale.

Worried Vicky will wake up and be furious I left, I quickly whisper the story into the phone. "Oh my God! What if she dies? I'm freaking out!"

"No. Don't freak out. She's just drunk," Nunnally insists. "But you shouldn't have to handle this—you're her *employee*. Just make her agree to go to the hospital."

Of course, he's right. Reluctantly, I go back and wait for her to rouse. "Vicky, please. I really think we should go to the hospital," I say when she does.

She squints up at me. "I'm your boss. And I'm telling you one final time: I'm *not* going to the hospital. Don't ask me again!" Her voice is furious and desperate, and I know with instant certainty that she's not going to die, she's just horribly drunk and she will do *anything* to avoid having a medical record of it.

As the hours wear on, we become an isolated island of oddness in a public setting. Women employees come in, pee in adjacent stalls, the liquid splashing sound loud in the silence, wash their hands, and leave. Each time someone walks out, I wish I could leave with her. Several offer us a doctor or a cab to the hospital, but each time, Vicky refuses all efforts. "We're fine!" she insists—a claim that resides somewhere between laughable and ludicrous when issued from someone lying next to a public toilet.

I mentally telegraph that we are *not* fine. That, in fact, it feels like my drunk boss is holding me hostage and I'm in desperate need of rescue. Surely, someone must see this isn't kosher. Surely someone will help me.

But no. I remain solo in my mission of getting Vicky cleaned up and presentable enough to get on a plane and back to Boston. I wish I had a copy of the employee handbook to consult. Would I look under "V" for "vomiting?" Or "D" for "drunk?" Or perhaps "C" for "crazy," and see if they have a subheading for "boss."

We miss our flight home.

"Call Betsy, get us on the next shuttle," Vicky croaks, eyes closed as though I'm tiring her out, as though she's not running up thousands of dollars in airline cancellation and rebooking fees.

Obediently, I relay the orders.

I sit and wait for Vicky to convey her readiness to leave. Naturally, we miss that flight as well.

Sweat rings appear under her armpits and around her neck and waist. "Get us on the seven."

Obediently, Betsy rebooks us yet again, her voice sympathetic. We're both powerless. I sit on the floor and answer emails while Vicky dozes fitfully.

"You like to take care of people," she says randomly. I'd mistakenly thought she was asleep.

I want to deny this. I don't like any part of this. I feel like a caged animal, trapped and helpless. I resent wasting an entire day sitting here as work piles up back at the office. I resent that I'm going to miss my yoga class and dinner with Nunnally. I resent that this woman is refusing to get medical help if she needs it and is wasting my time if she doesn't.

But how do you say that to your new boss? Your new boss who's in charge of your year-end evaluation? Your new boss who controls whether you receive the year-end bonus you've been promised? Being the fortuitous possessor of an intellect roughly equivalent to sheer, unmitigated genius, I know I shouldn't have to handle this situation alone. But I *don't* know how to extricate myself without angering said boss. So in spite of my misgivings, I continue sitting beside her. I continue taking care of her. I continue asking solicitously if there's anything she needs. But most of all, I continue pretending that this somehow isn't an unmitigated, code-red disaster. That this isn't, in fact, the craziest, most fucked-up day on the job—any job—that I've ever had.

Eventually, I get Vicky downstairs and into a cab. She opens the window and stares out as we weave through rush-hour traffic to La Guardia. "Take care of it," she snaps over her shoulder as soon as we pull up to the terminal. Obediently, I pay the driver and wrestle our luggage to the gate.

Although Betsy booked us seats on the plane that were nowhere near each other—I wonder fleetingly if this was an act of mercy or an unintended result of the last-minute rebooking—Vicky demands the flight attendant procure us seats together in case she becomes sick again. Ushered to our new adjacent location, she claims the aisle seat and promptly passes out, her head lolling forward. I fantasize briefly about smashing her forehead into the tray table and playing it off like she did it to herself, but resist.

We land and Vicky strides ahead as I manage all the bags to the curb.

She climbs in the town car that Betsy has waiting for us and turns to me. "Are you going in to the office now?"

I look at the time—8:30 pm. Is she joking? "No."

"No?" she echoes mockingly, one eyebrow rocketing up. I've never dared to openly disobey her. She makes it clear I'll pay for this later. "Well, I am. We've wasted a whole day and we have a lot of work to do. By the way, clear your schedule tomorrow morning—I have an acting lesson so you need to go evaluate entertainment acts for our next conference." She yanks the door shut and is gone, leaving me standing on the airport sidewalk, freezing and alone in the cold December night.

Chapter Four

The Bad Boss Blues

The next morning, I wake up early and make my way downtown to the theater district, where a small theater is hosting the performer showcase. I slip quietly into a seat in the sparsely populated orchestra section and yawn. By the time I'd gotten home last night, ordered in dinner, and poured out the whole story in excruciating detail to Nunnally, it had made for another late night. Still though, there was something so therapeutic about relating it all to him. I wasn't sure if it was the fact that he loved me, his comforting lawyerliness, or something intrinsically soothing about this man, but I simply had to tell him every single detail of my day, especially when it was a crazy one. It was the mental equivalent of wiping down the counters before I went to bed; I couldn't rest without completing the ritual.

A series of performers queue up to go onstage and I refocus my attention, trying not to think about the work that's piling up by the nanosecond back at the office. I rate dancers, jugglers, several comedians, motivational speakers, and a few bands. I take two sets of notes—one for Vicky, henceforth to be known as Vomiting Vicky, and one to keep myself entertained. *Demonstrates the core Investorcap value of commitment to professional development/I've heard screeching cats sound better. A strong value-add/this a-hole will fit right in.*

Quiet laughter to my right makes me jerk guiltily.

A dark-haired guy I hadn't noticed sitting next to me points to my "Vomiting Vicky" column header. "Must be pretty bad." His voice is warm and conspiratorial.

"No...they were okay...I'm just being harsh," I lie defensively, blushing furiously.

He laughs again. "No, I mean where you work. Or who you work *for*...."

"You have no idea," I say, laughing too.

"Paul Johnson," he says, confidently extending a hand. "And I'm actually auditioning later. I hope you'll be kinder in your eval of me."

"I'm Sara, and I should probably skip last names and other identifying details."

He laughs. "If I'd known we were using code names, I would've used my stage name, Sweet Pauley."

Sweet Pauley turns out to be extraordinarily nice. Even better, he works as a life coach, and, taking pity on me after what he correctly imagines is a challenging workplace situation, offers to give me a coaching session later that week. I'm thrilled to accept, but spend the next several days wondering what I'll say.

The appointed day arrives. After work, I head to the agreed upon cafe and find Sweet Pauley sitting casually with one leg crossed on his knee. Blushing, I mumble an awkward hello, as I wonder if this was all a big mistake, and take the seat opposite him.

He simply looks at me, quietly knowing, as we sit in expectant silence. Finally, in the intimacy born of talking to a stranger, I say, "So I guess it's pretty clear that I hate what I do." Immediately, overwhelming guilt for that admission sweeps in. Who am I to complain? I'm lucky to have a job. I quickly temper the truth with an upbeat, "But, hey, who doesn't, right?"

He ignores this attempt. "Why do you do it then?"

I shrug. "The usual reasons—student loans, mortgage, car payments…."

"And what do you love in your life?"

"Well…I have a great boyfriend. I love him."

He nods. "Yeah, I have a great boyfriend too. But relationships are a separate category. You can't rely on anyone or anything outside yourself for your happiness. We're going to talk today about doing something for yourself. About taking time for yourself to do something that's only yours…that brings you happiness. So, what do *you* do for *you*?"

"*Me?*" My tone clearly conveys that that's a ludicrous question—that taking time to do something for myself isn't an option.

But Sweet Pauley ignores my tone. He continues watching me, quiet and serious.

"Well...I do yoga twice a week. That's for me." I offer this up to him.

He isn't distracted by this offering. "Sara, everyone deserves—no, *needs*—something that's just for themselves. More than yoga twice a week. What do you *really* want? What would make you happier?"

"I could go more often?" Why am I asking him?

"You need more than just more classes. Your job's weighing this side down," he says, holding his hands up like the scales of justice and lowering one. "So you need more on this side to balance it." He brings his hands back to equilibrium. "Make it a field project. Explore what you want to do. There must be other ways to expand yoga, like trainings or something. You obviously love it."

I nod. "Well, there are teacher trainings. But I never even considered them because I would never be a yoga teacher. I mean...that would be ridiculous." I roll my eyes and pause long enough to let him know there's no two ways about that. Yoga teachers are Zen-looking, ethereal, vegan creatures who float around emanating wisdom. I look down at my pinstriped navy blue suit and gleaming patent leather heels, and smile at the incongruity. "But I guess I could just go to...you know, improve and advance."

Still looking at me as though he sees through to my soul, he nods.

Brain buzzing, I walk out of the cafe. *What do I want? What can I do just for myself?* The questions are tantalizing. Terrifying. Overwhelming. Who has the time to ponder these sorts of things? Who has the luxury of thinking about what they *want* to do? And who the hell is this Sweet Pauley guy anyway?

In the cherished type-A American game of who can work the hardest, be the most stressed out, have little or no time for themselves, and proudly display the ill effects of a job that is consuming them, I am winning. Of course I hate my job—

everyone hates their job…or so I tell myself. But there's nothing I can do about it. There are bills and loans and mortgages to pay. There isn't enough bandwidth to step back and *think*, and even if there was, I couldn't do anything about it.

Unless…there was and I could?

My brain hurts as the seemingly ironclad lines I live within sway and blur. I shake my head firmly. I need to escape to a class to disentangle the thoughts racing around my brain, to focus on a plan. As always, my mat is soothing in its familiarity, in its promise of renewal. I smile and wave at a few yoga buddies. In attendance tonight is the usual bevy of Back Bay beauties—young, slender, and well dressed. My friends Isabella and Julie, who I'd met in class a few years ago, join me in our usual spot. We chat idly before the teacher arrives and we zealously dive in.

But this night, I'm distracted. In the years since I'd started, naturally I'd gotten better—stronger, suppler, more familiar with the poses. I no longer had to concentrate fiercely to understand the names or mechanics—my body flowed knowingly through the series. The downside of this is that it gives my brain plenty of time to wander. I step forward to warrior one. *Am I being impractical? Maybe I should just keep trying to brace up like my Italian Nana always says.* In downward-facing dog, I argue that I've already wasted years bracing up. *If not now, then when?* I volley silently back. I mentally debate this for the next 90 minutes. Finally, in s*avasana,* physically spent, demons as tamed as they're going to get, I admit that as much as I love doing yoga—and as much salvation as each class provides—it's still not enough to counterbalance my job. Sweet Pauley's right.

But yoga teacher training might be. And, as tonight's class had proved, I needed a new challenge. A training would allow me to get better at something I loved, and, more importantly, serve as a substantial entity in my life that wasn't my job or relationship. It would, as Sweet Pauley had said, be something just for me.

Sure, not all the classes I've taken have been as magical as that first daring dip when I was nursing a broken heart, but overall, something had clicked deep within me, and that initial recognition had blossomed into a nurturing and sustaining practice on the mat. That practice had stayed with me through changes in address, jobs, and relationships that yielded additional heartbreak. Especially my last one, before meeting Nunnally, which had ended in the crushing discovery of his cheating on me with his assistant.

I'd been thinking about the possibility of someday taking a training for almost as long as I'd been practicing. But, you know, only thinking about it in the margins of my mind, because to really think about it was too impractical, something for other people, not an option for me. But now Sweet Pauley was telling me to explore.

I tell Nunnally about the field project. "You should definitely do it," he says.

"But isn't it…I don't know…self-indulgent?"

"There's a big difference between having something for yourself and being *self-indulgent*. You should do it."

I smile, already excited.

Several days, many online searches, and one cross-referenced spreadsheet later, I find Tri Dosha Yoga. Under the direction of its founder, Theadosia (Thea) Taylor, the program is more impressive than anything else I've ever heard about. It includes instruction from a professor at a local university on anatomy and physiology, various workshops in therapeutically addressing chronic conditions and injuries, extensive written work, group and individual projects, and supervised work as an assistant in Thea's own classes. Thea herself is just as impressive, with a slew of degrees, including a PhD in psychology and decades of experience in the field. Naturally, she also holds the highest level of yoga certifications available as well…from no less than three different schools of yoga. When she's not running this program or teaching, she tours internationally, speaking at conferences and training teachers.

The thoroughness and professionalism of the program, the exacting nature of its requirements, and the prospect of training under Thea's direct supervision is thrilling.

The Tri Dosha Yoga philosophy of tending to each individual body resonates with me; other programs seem so generic. I can't believe my good fortune that this renowned program is held in New Hampshire, only an hour away from Boston. I immediately fill out the online contact request form to set up a phone interview.

When Thea herself calls me a few days later, I'm excited and intimidated to talk with her. I tell her I like her focus on modifying poses to fit different students' needs, rather than forcing the body to fit the pose. "I also like your import-an-expert concept. That seems like a competitive differentiator for your program."

She laughs gently. "Wow! You really know marketing!"

I smile. It's endearing that she's impressed by a passing reference to a basic marketing concept. Meanwhile, she holds a PhD and travels the world as a teacher of teachers. She's renowned and I'm a faceless corporate drone, but I guess I *do* know PR and marketing, even if I don't like it. "So…I've already checked out your website," I say, leaving out that I've printed every page, gone through each section with color-coded highlighters, and pretty much memorized it. "What would you say is the most important thing I should know about your program?"

She laughs gently as though my organization and attention to detail are sweet. "Well, let's see…our school focuses on the exploration of the mind-body aspects of yoga and the potential to rewire the neuro-structure of the brain and nervous system. It's a chance for practitioners to equalize imbalances of neuro-emotional states such as anxiety and depression. We believe that the possibility for healing and change is innate within each of us, that we all hold the keys to our evolution." Her voice is like a song. Her words are brilliant and hypnotic.

Having practiced for seven years, I'd already felt in my own body yoga's calming and strengthening effects. However, Thea, with a doctorate to back it up, was talking about the therapeutic applications of yoga…about possibilities I hadn't even heard of in the "mind-body" realm—something I also hadn't heard of.

I hesitantly ask if there's room left for enrollment, holding my breath.

"There are a few more spots available," Thea warmly assures me. "I encourage you to apply if this feels like a good fit."

We get off the phone and I restrain myself—barely—from jumping around like a hyper little primate, screaming "It's the *perfect fit! Perfect fit!*" In a corporate-instilled involuntary tic, I glance at the timer on my phone and realize we've talked for over half an hour. By any measure, this is a generous amount of her time. I'm honored that Thea has made time to talk to me in her international-touring-teaching-important-person schedule. Her syllabus doesn't include the yoga world staples of chanting or meditation, but this only convinces me of her brilliance. She doesn't adhere to tradition; she's an innovator.

Although I desperately want to be part of this training, I'm intimidated by Thea's status, her education, and the depth of her knowledge. Wondering if I'll even get in, I begin filling out the lengthy application. I pause when I get to the list of requirements; one is that all trainees are supposed to be "drug-free," which is defined as tobacco-, caffeine-, and alcohol-free (also presumably heroin-, cocaine-, and meth-free but I don't plan to ask) as of the first day of training. Vegetarianism is "strongly encouraged."

I've never smoked and never will, so that's not a problem. But I think of the fancy coffeemaker at work with options like Belgian chocolate and Rio dark that I enjoy multiple times per day. I think of the wine I enjoy over dinner or after a stressful day. I think of the gin and tonics that my friend Leigh and I love to make on hot summer nights while we barbeque nonvegetarian food on her patio. What's the harm in these yoga violations? And really…how would they know if I wasn't fully adhering?

I mentally slap myself. It's on the honor system, this being yoga and all, and I shouldn't even be thinking of how to con the system. If these are the rules, I should comply, even if it seems a bit extreme not to enjoy these small pleasures. I'm already at enough of a disadvantage as everyone else will probably be *über*-advanced. I imagine gorgeous, skinny, super-yoginis twisted up in crazy circus-like pretzel poses. Poses I've never been able to execute and probably never will.

Self-consciously, I forge ahead. But when I get to the question about what poses are most challenging, I chew my lip and hesitate to answer honestly. I want to say, "Um…do you want that alphabetically or in descending order?" But insecurity prompts me to fill in "arm balances" instead.

Several more pages, including questions on any injuries or mental illness (*um...none?*), and finally it's complete. Feeling boldly adventurous and totally insecure, I put the stack into a folder marked "Field Project" and lock it in one of my cabinets, safe from the probing eyes of inquisitive colleagues. I float on the current of hope for a few excited hours.

Not long after, however, the shadowy, insidious figure of doubt enters my brain, followed swiftly by overwhelming guilt. As hard as I work, Nunnally works even harder. A big-firm lawyer yoked to the unenviable weight of billable hour requirements and an unrelenting workload, he never leaves the office before eight pm and usually it's later. Nights and weekends mean nothing—his Blackberry bleats at him incessantly, whereas mine only bleats every so often if I don't "accidentally" leave it at the office in a desperate attempt to have work-life separation. That separation is a luxury Nunnally's never allowed. When he's not at the office, he still spends most of his time in front of his laptop, working. He pulls at least one all-nighter a month and he rarely complains.

I, on the other hand, have never had to pull an all-nighter. So as much as my job sucks, and while I indisputably deal with more bitches, intraoffice politics, and bullshit, Nunnally has to deal with corporate bullshit—and *still* works at least double what I do. All of which leads me to the inescapable conclusion that I'm a loser for complaining. In comparison, I have a pretty great job. Heck, I'm lucky have a job at all—I recognize that many aren't as fortunate.

My job has also enabled me to be a major financial contributor to my relationship, buy an apartment, theoretically pay for my dream of seeing the world a little bit at a time—which the generous vacation policy of four weeks per year also allows for (even though I never actually use it), save for my retirement, and buy fun little things whenever I want to, extravagances I'd scarcely dreamed of growing up as I did, poor and living in hand-me-downs from my cousins.

Most important, unlike ridiculous, deplorable, and ultimately sad Vicky, I have a life outside of work: a yoga practice that sustains me, revives me, and keeps me fit; fantastic friends; wonderful family members; and, to top it all off, Nunnally. To ask for more is just plain ungrateful. I'm ashamed. What the hell was I thinking? Who did I think I was? What made me think I was entitled to ask—to even dare to think of greedily asking for more? I resolve to forget about this whole training thing.

Chapter Five
Captain Theatrical Runs Aground

Tue to my plan, I "brace up" for the next few months and manage, with some success, to fly stealth under Vomiting Vicky's radar. There isn't any more vomit or caretaking on bathroom floors, but there's been plenty of other sorts of work-place adventures, and, while less acidic than vomit, the outcome was ultimately just as corrosive. In a nutshell, I continue to fight every day to keep from drowning in the cesspool of my professional life.

There have been just enough positives to buoy me up, the net result keeping my head just barely above water. There was the challenge of my work—building a PR program, the rigors of which certainly provided plenty of distraction. There was the encouragement that other people at least seemed to think I was good at my job—I was nominated (albeit most certainly not by Vicky) for the Most Valuable Employee Award and came in second. There was my yoga practice—sacred pockets of time where I breathed out my tension and stretched out my desk-jockey muscles.

Perhaps most important, there was the wonderful personal life distraction of getting engaged to Nunnally. This heralded the welcome relief that my 95-year-old Italian Nana no longer had to introduce me as "the unmarried one." Because, you know, at the ripe old age of 29, it was a crime against Italian humanity that I remained stubbornly single.

As my 29th birthday passes, the self-imposed countdown to 30 that most 20-somethings subject themselves to intensifies. I'd been dreading turning 30 practically since the day I'd turned 20. Thirty was the age by which I had always imagined that I'd have everything figured out. I'd have my dream job. In the city (which city didn't matter at the time). And I'd have fabulous outfits. The pinnacle of which, I envisioned, would be knee-high leather boots and a just above-the-knee skirt. In this ensemble, I would stride down sunny sidewalks (it was always sunny in these daydreams), in a haze of happiness due in equal measure to my dream job and killer wardrobe.

In reality, 30 is creeping closer and I still feel completely lost, working in a field that I'm not only completely *uninterested* in, but also actively *loathe*, under an attention-grabbing, wine-guzzling banshee who actively loathes *me* in return. Not even yoga can change that.

Gathering my budding courage, I send resumes for every nonprofit job I can find. I figure that, in spite of the scary pay cut, I can at least explore starting a new decade in a more meaningful area.

I receive only one response: an auto-generated reply telling me they'll contact me if they're interested. *Yeah…they don't.*

Meanwhile, financial services recruiters chase me. But I've learned from the last change that I need to escape the finance world altogether, that I want to actually *help* people. I confide this to one recruiter and she cheerily informs me that I missed that window—I'm now pigeon-holed in the finance industry. I thank her and hang up.

I send more resumes. I'm met only with resounding silence in response. As the weeks pass, hope slowly shrivels and eventually dies. I feel rejected, unwanted, and very, very trapped.

Things aren't getting any better at work. Plummeting into what surely must be clinical paranoia, Vicky starts to imagine that the company is maneuvering against her ascension to Executive Vice President. She starts to find fault with everything— from what I wear to what Betsy and the other admins wear. She makes me stay late one Friday night to meet with her. Nervously, I watch the clock as I wait to be summoned to her office.

My sisters, Annie and Hanna, are flying in tonight and staying for the weekend for an overdue visit and to begin apartment hunting. Annie, who just finished her master's degree, and Hanna, who just completed her bachelor's, have been roommates in North Carolina since Hanna was old enough to go to college and selected the same school Annie was already attending. Their age difference worked perfectly for graduating together with their respective degrees. Now, they were planning to move to Boston to be closer to me and because, like me, they liked the prospect of a smaller city with easy beach and mountain access, not to mention a plentiful job market (even if it wasn't the jobs I wanted).

Finally, Vicky calls me. I pray this will be quick so I can get home and do some desperately needed cleaning before heading to the airport to pick up my sisters.

"We're here to talk about your rebellion," Vicky says as soon as I'm seated. "I know you're plotting a mutiny to rise up, overthrow me, and steal my job."

I stare, dumbfounded. Then my brain kicks into gear. "What? That's crazy! I would never do that! I would never even think to do that!" (And honestly, I hadn't. Which is too bad, because if I had thought of it, I really might have tried as a measure of self-preservation.)

"You are! You are! I know you are!" She's sweating, pacing, frenzied.

I feel a shiver of genuine fear. I glance furtively toward the door. My mind spins. If only I'd been there longer, if only I knew someone in human resources I could confide in. But I have neither of these. Vicky's been here for over ten years. She's been retained and promoted. Although it's unfathomable to me, they seem to value and trust her.

In contrast, I'm relatively new and, in a word, screwed.

She slams her palms on the armrests of my chair and leans in menacingly. I feel her breath on my face. She stares me down.

I shrink into the chair, retreating into silence. Anything to end this interaction and get out of here, home, and safely into the weekend. I need to redouble my resume-sending efforts. In case it wasn't crystal clear before, it is now: Mama needs a new job.

"Even the way you sit there is rebellious! I'm on to you and don't think I'm not!" She jabs her finger at me. Her rage is intense, intimidating.

I sit frozen, looking into her crazed eyes for what feels like an eternity. Finally, she flings her hands off the armrests of my chair and points silently to the door, breathing heavily. I scurry out of her office.

Shaking, I quickly collect my bag from my office and rush out of the building. I hurry home, dreading ever having to return and simultaneously terrified of being fired. As I climb the stairs toward our fifth-floor apartment, my cell phone rings. I shudder—Vicky? HR? But no, it's my future mother-in-law. I let it roll to voicemail as I unlock the door, drop my workbag, and kick off my heels. Moments later, I don sweatpants and start dusting the bookshelves. Rows of yoga manuals, cookbooks, and travel guides—three on India alone—look down at me. These are symbols of my aspirational life, where I deepen my knowledge of yoga, cook elaborate meals, and travel through Southeast Asia.

I ignore them and yank open the Ikea wardrobe that serves as a closet in our tiny apartment that has no closets, and pull out the vacuum. The small size of this apartment can be most accurately conveyed by how long it takes to vacuum (five minutes) and how many times you have to plug in the cord in order to reach it all (one). I aspire to someday live in an apartment large enough that it will actually require unplugging and re-plugging the vacuum multiple times. My dream home will also have a guest room. As it is, I can reach every corner from one centralized outlet and my sisters sleep on an air mattress on the floor.

A text message pings. "Honey, are you free for a bridesmaid dress appointment tomorrow at noon?"

I grit my teeth and put the vacuum away. In his lawyerly, diplomatic way, Nunnally had recently alerted me to the fact that his mom doesn't consider the J. Crew dresses that all the bridesmaids have already purchased "traditional enough." To help her feel included in the wedding process, he asked me to spend a day looking at more conventional options with her. I don't have to change dresses if I don't want to, he clarified, it would just be nice to consider it so she feels included. *Great. Just what I want to do on my day off.*

At the same time, I do want her to feel included, especially since the mother of the groom is usually excluded and she only had sons. It was also my only chance at motherly involvement, the lack of which I'd felt acutely during this wedding-planning process. Aside from Mother's Day every year, I'd never felt more mother-less than while wedding planning.

Regardless of feelings of exclusion and motherly participation, I don't have the luxury of wasting time on wedding tasks, *especially* ones that I've already checked off the list. I can't even spend time helping my sisters look for apartments. And while it's sad that anything outside of work feels like "wasted" time, that's the reality of working a demanding job. And right now I need to buckle down and use the weekend to look for a new demanding job. There isn't another option. I need to tire-lessly crank the wheel to get myself the hell out of Investorcap and far away from Vicky.

But I can't do that either. I just *can't*. I'm so worn down from the job itself, and evading Vicky's histrionics and the crushing failure of my most recent job search, that even the prospect of further job hunting—every tiny step of that process—seems entirely overwhelming.

When you work a stressful, fast-paced corporate job and spend your entire day putting out fires, trying to cram a week's worth of work into each day…and then you layer on top of that someone who drives the very spirit out of you, the idea of com-ing home from five consecutive days of that and somehow summoning up the ener-gy—even the mental *will*—to put yourself out there for rejection yet again, is so completely and utterly overwhelming…so absolutely *exhausting* that it renders the idea simply impossible. It renders the idea of doing anything other than flopping on the couch and reaching for the wine impossible. Even yoga—my escape and my sol-ace—is too much effort to consider.

I'm ashamed of my mental inertia, but truthfully, the familiarity of dysfunction seems less exhausting than the idea, let alone the action, of finding and moving on to something new.

Feelings of guilt for having a good-paying job and yet still wanting to be free of said job, as well as my innate determination to make any situation work, no matter how crazy or bad, smolder beneath my feelings of desperation and resentment. Layered on top of that is my fear that I'd leapt only further into the fire with my last job change. I shudder to think where I might land next.

The weekend flies by in a blur of compulsive job searching intermingled with helping my sisters look for apartments (of course I couldn't let them go alone no matter how crunched I was for time) and the requisite bridesmaid dress excursion. After trying on every single bridesmaid option the store offered, I'd shrugged helplessly and concluded that unfortunately I wanted to stay with my original choice. It was a successful endeavor nonetheless: Nunnally's mom felt included, and I'd gotten a taste of motherly involvement.

I go into the office early Monday. I want to get settled before Vicky arrives. Weirdly, there's already a voicemail waiting from human resources asking me to "stop by at my earliest convenience." This is the most bone-chilling message a corporate person can receive. I immediately rush down to the HR wing—scarily secluded behind an additional security door—wondering what's going on. A relatively junior HR associate sternly informs me that Vicky has submitted a litany of complaints against me including "insubordination." This is to serve as a written warning. Apparently, Vicky's mutiny accusation constituted a "verbal warning."

I stumble back to my office. It's somewhere between shocking and humiliating to be on the receiving end of a complaint regarding professionalism from a drunken lunatic vomiter. Despite my comparatively newly hired status, I decide I won't just slink off into a corner. I respond with a written complaint of my own, refuting all of Vicky's claims and filling them in on her drunkenness, botched presentation in New York, and paranoid tirades.

Apparently, that's all it takes to get heard. Minutes after I click "send," the head of HR asks to meet. She's a woman known for her substantial size, her even-larger platinum-blond perm, and her omnipresent cowboy boots in varying colors. The scent of her perfume is overwhelming. I try not to be distracted by it as she grills me about every detail: dates, times, client witnesses, etc. Finally, she stands. "We'll look into it, but I can't tell you anything. Confidentiality, you know." She shakes my hand and I leave her office and the HR wing for the second time that morning.

I go back to my desk. Am I actually supposed to keep working? How can I think about anything except what's going to happen next? My brain spins frantically as the day crawls by. *Maybe things will get better. Maybe Vomiting Vicky will be fired! If she is, maybe I should stay here because, despite its meaninglessness, I'm good at this job and it pays well. If she's not fired, I'll definitely have to leave. So which one of us will it be? Her or me? Will she even know a complaint's been filed against her? Were they investigating her already? Where will that leave me then?*

I see Vicky only once as she walks by my office. She ignores me. My anxiety ratchets up. If she finds out about the responsorial HR Armageddon I've unleashed against her, things are going to get even less chummy than they were on the bathroom floor during the Great Upchuck Incident.

I rub my forehead. I've been in high-stress, hyper-vigilant mode for far too many long-ass years. The chronic stress, tight deadlines, and excessive, unnecessary travel have systematically broken me down. Even the need to always be on guard, keeping up the daily pretense that I'm interested in the work I do, that I believe in these products and this industry is stealthily erosive. The simple truth is that continuous posturing to keep up these pretenses is psychically exhausting. There is also the small matter of having a code-red crazy for a boss. So far, it's been manageable. *Barely.* But now, tipping the scale in favor of a total freaking meltdown, I have the shadow of the big 3-0 hulking over me like a giant grim reaper and the never-ending process of wedding planning riding me like Seabiscuit.

Maybe back when I was in my first job, I could keep slogging through this corporate sludge, the luck of having a job and the luxury of being able to make a decent living enough to keep me going indefinitely.

But I'm not in my first job. I've waded in deep enough that I am, as the recruiter pointed out, solidly pigeon holed. The prospect of remaining stuck here for who-knows-how-much longer relentlessly chips away at the deepest part of me. Like moving water washes unremittingly over jagged rocks, eventually wearing them down until they're rounded and smooth, time in this business has been wearing me down, insidiously eroding the very spirit and individuality that makes me, *me*. The inauthenticity of my daily existence, coupled with forcing myself to remain in said existence, has cleaved huge chunks out of my sense of self.

I feel as though the treacherous undertow of my daily life, of these daily deceptions, washes me ever further from the shoreline of escape and safety, where my truth, whatever it is, resides, and where the next chapter, whatever it holds, will begin.

Accustomed to living just under the boiling point but now decidedly boiling over after the fabricated insubordination complaint, there is only one place to turn. Desperate and low, I crave the solace of my yoga practice.

I log on to the Tri Dosha Yoga website. My completed application remains in the cabinet right above my head, a dormant seed that I'd never allowed myself to plant.

Ignoring its nearness, I see that Thea, as luck would have it, is teaching in Boston tonight. At the stroke of five, I grab the spare mat I keep under the desk, and rush to the elevator, not speaking to anyone, not even making eye contact. I'm single-minded in focusing on escape. I need the sanctuary of my yoga practice and I want to experience Thea's teaching for myself, without any special attention.

I hurry through the streets until I'm practically running. As I enter the hushed lobby, I take note of the carefully selected pieces of driftwood designed to look incidentally scattered about.

"Welcome. May I offer you an organic, *ayurvedically* balancing cup of tea as you check in?" a smiling woman wearing a kimono-inspired uniform asks. Her posh, composed manner matches this place.

I pay the $24 without question, and she presses a eucalyptus-steamed "refreshment" towel into my hands as she escorts me to the women's "rejuvenation zone," known in lesser establishments as the locker room. I stuff my work bag into a bamboo locker, change, and hurry down the hall, wondering if I've entered the luxury twilight zone of the yoga world.

Chapter Six

Hello Yoga? It's Me…Again

I take a long, slow breath at the classroom door and try to leave Vicky, HR, and the rest of my day here, outside. Maybe next to the fruit-infused mineral water bar. My galloping thoughts are like a runaway stagecoach in an old western. *Stop thinking about work,* I tell myself. *Seriously, just stop.*

I push the heavy wooden door open, place my mat in the back row, and look around, feeling every inch a country mouse. Apparently, I've checked in to the Ritz Carlton of yoga venues. The fact that my gym even attempts to have a yoga room now seems like a sad little joke. This place is like a luxurious spa. And for 24 bucks a class, that seems appropriate. The space is dim and intimate, lit only by the soft glow of candles. The bamboo floors are stained a deep shade of gleaming brown; a serene Buddha perches at the front. There are floor-to-ceiling curtains in an exquisite, rich turquoise at the back. Behind them are shelves full of fresh new bolsters, blankets, blocks, and straps. I take none of these—the classes I take don't use props and I take a certain level of pride in that.

It's a small class, only about 12 mats are scattered around the room. Atop them rest a slightly more luxe version of the Back Bay beauties who frequent my regular, equally clean but more basic gym. All are slender. All are manicured and pedicured. Various shades of perfectly coiffed hair are highlighted and lowlighted to peak expensive perfection. Everyone is wearing some version of $100 yoga pants and color-coordinated tops. I feel underdressed…in a yoga class.

The door opens, and a hush falls over the room as Thea glides in. Reflexively, I draw an excited, nervous breath. An ethereal pixie of a person, Thea is delicate and lithe. She stands about five feet three inches and has fine, pale blond hair that wisps about her face in a short, shaggy cut. She looks like a cross between Twiggy, the famous 1960s model, and Madonna, who Thea just might be able to beat in a yoga arm wrestling match. Impressively defined arms aside, Thea seems somehow not of this world. She reminds me of a mischievous winged fairy I saw once in a children's book. All she needs is a tutu and a wand and I'm sure she could sprout some wings. She's one of those people whose age is impossible to define, but based on her academic and professional accomplishments alone, I'd place her somewhere in her mid-fifties.

Thea welcomes new people and asks about injuries before announcing that everyone will need props. Feeling a tad miffed—*props are for losers, duh*—I nonetheless go to retrieve them.

We begin kneeling in *virasana*, hero's pose, "Let's begin by with our drop in," Thea says in a way that makes me think we'll be here for a while, even though I don't know what the "drop in" is. I push away the smug thought that I'm used to diving right in.

The first thing I notice is the silence, the stillness. Having started in the *ashtanga* tradition, also a silent practice, but then later diversified with *vinyasa* classes, which are often practiced to music, I'd gotten used to the distraction that music could provide—the background noise, the mental cushion from the ping-ponging of my thoughts.

Now, here, there was silence again. But it wasn't the same sort of silence as my *ashtanga* classes—it wasn't an intense penetrating silence pregnant with the impending promise of strenuous physical activity. *Ashtanga* silence is also tinged with the competitive nature innate in power yoga classes—where, in my experience, pushing yourself to your physical limits, or even a bit beyond, is expected and encouraged. But neither was this the passive, idle silence of the mindless sort of classes that I sometimes drop into by chance at the gym, which pretty much amount to half-assed-*asana*.

Although I'd never before been conscious of the variations and intensities of silence—in fact, I'd never really thought about silence at all—I notice immediately that something about *this* silence is different. It's active and present, calm and controlled. It doesn't just loll there, existing because of a lack of sound—because eventually there is sound as Thea introduces *ujjiy*, victorious breathing, and then the silence becomes richer as it's punctuated with the chug-chug of the class's *ujjiy* pulse.

No, this silence is different because it is here intentionally, under the orchestration, management, and direction of Thea as the teacher, the conductor. There's also a certain dynamic vitality to the silence—to the space in the room—an energy, a magnetic field-like sphere that I can't see but can definitely feel. There, dancing just beyond the peripheries of awareness, is a certain, dare I say...*spirituality?*

And it felt daring to think this, because it seems that to speak of spirituality is so very...*passé*, so totally uncool, so completely dorky. Sadly, it seems that the only people who speak of spirituality, faith, or religion are either fanatics or New Agers—and let's be honest, neither of those groups are known for their normalcy, let alone cool factors. The fact is that yoga is predominantly a physical practice in the US, and any spiritual aspects have remained unknown to me.

Back in the moment, I'm simply curious to see where this 90-minute journey will go. And without thinking about why or how, I know it feels safe to be here. It feels safe to release my never-ending need to be watching, observing, and guarding. Thea's at the helm of this expedition, and I'm in good and capable hands.

Usually, even when I'm a passenger in a car, I still feel the need to be as alert as if I were actually driving—after all, if I'm not there to anxiously read street signs, keep us on track, and compulsively make sure we don't miss a turn, how can I ensure we'll arrive? But something about Thea's presence makes it clear that she's going to handle everything, and so I rearrange my mental analogy: this is more like being on a plane—I know they're not going to let me help the pilot (unfortunately), so I just sit back and try to relax. (Or, in my case, sit back and nervously clutch the armrests, hoping the plane won't go down in a fiery crash.)

In this room, in this practice, I feel but can't explain how Thea is both creating and guiding the space—that the silence exists because of her. That the silence is a tool that she's using for purposes unknown to me, and that it has levels, tones, and richness to it because she intends it to be that way. I follow her guiding voice during the drop-in and feel myself falling into it like a pillow. My shoulders go slack and my face relaxes. As though someone unplugged the power cord to my stress source or handed me a giant class of sauvignon blanc, my whole body loosens.

Is this meditation? I wonder. Whatever it is, I'm slinging it back faster than a frat boy at an open bar.

We emerge and she leads us through breathwork, *pranayama*, blocking alternating nostrils and inhaling and exhaling through only one at a time. This too is...different, but I emerge feeling relaxed. I like this drop-in thing, but can't help wondering what the active practice will look like after such a long intro. *Will I get a good workout?*

About ten minutes later, I'm glad we did the drop in for as long as we had and wonder if I might request a longer one next time. In spite, or perhaps because, of the fact that we move slowly—more slowly than in any class I'd ever taken, and in fact more slowly than I've ever moved before at all—it's quickly apparent that this is one of the most challenging practices I've ever done. As we hold and micro-adjust each pose, my legs shake to support my weight and my breath stops altogether.

This is something I haven't felt since I first started practicing. Eventually, my body acclimated to the *ashtanga* method—abdominal and arm muscle definition appeared for the first time in my life, my overall strength increased, my balance improved...in short, my body stepped up to meet the demands I'd placed on it.

And so, for some time now, yoga has no longer felt very challenging compared to my first class when it was all I could do just to get through. Now, the poses, their Sanskrit names, the flow, and order were familiar to me. I was comfortable and confident enough that my monkey-chatter brain had even resumed its ceaseless barking.

But this class is another beast entirely. We hold the poses so long my leg screams for release, then we shift to another pose for an eternity...weight still on that one quivering leg. Then Thea reminds us firmly to check in with our breath, or deepen our breath, to use our breath to explore "latent parts" of ourselves. I feel like a beginner again.

I'm profoundly grateful for the support of the props I'd been so reluctant to get at the beginning. Based on the fact that she'd asked for requests, each Tri Dosha class is customized to the needs of the students. This is distinctly different from *ashtanga,* where the sequence is always the same—same poses, same order. Over the years, I'd found this comforting. As with the rest of my life, I liked knowing what to expect. But eventually, this repetition had started to feel stagnant.

Which led to a sort of awe of Thea's on-the-fly sequencing. How did she design something that felt so right, without planning, and have it all flow and come together so perfectly?

Additionally, and perhaps most importantly, there is another element of Thea's language that permeates the class atmosphere that I can't name—but can only describe as a level of depth and richness. Surely it must be a spiritual aspect. Even though she never speaks directly of it, talks about it, or preaches…it exists here all the same.

This isn't just a physical practice. And I like that.

Thea closes with three communal chants of "OM." This too is something new, as the classes I regularly attend don't chant. The other students raise their voices, and the class harmonizes effortlessly. It's more than beautiful—it feels good.

As the last "mmmm" leaves my chest and lingers in the air, Thea speaks. "Feeling the deep, powerful vibration of OM within you and carrying it with you to your practice off the mat…*namaste.*"

She bows her head and the class is finished.

My brain glows calmly. *My practice off the mat.* To view life through two lenses: on the mat and off, instead of at work and not at work. And what about viewing *life* as a *practice. Practice?* I wasn't even used to talking about yoga as a "practice," let alone life. Like almost everyone I know, there's nothing practice-y about life. I take life seriously—sort of like a competitive sport. I have to go, do, try, achieve, and fret over it all in my spare moments. *Practice?* An interesting concept.

I leave with a whole-hearted contentment that is a deeper, richer, and fuller experience than the sheer physical exhaustion of power yoga or the full, but rather unsatisfying, *vinyasas* I've taken—kind of like when I think it'll be fun to have ice cream for dinner, then feel full but not *fed*. This, however, felt deeply nourishing, like a Thanksgiving meal lovingly prepared.

It's like I'm falling in love with yoga all over again. I'd never been in a relationship long enough to experience what seasoned couples had always told me: every relationship ebbs and flows over time. You're never going to feel intense love every day for anyone or anything. Winter will come. Love might hibernate, and you'll wonder if it's gone forever, plummeting into doubt that it's ever coming back. But then spring arrives, whether it's in the calendar seasons or the seasons of long-lasting relationships, and suddenly the feelings bloom brightly again. Father Bob, the priest who's going to marry us, once said the same about his relationship with God.

This yoga relationship has been, by far, my longest. And to be fair, it's always been rather one-sided. Yoga gives and I take—comfort, stress relief, stretching, strengthening. Lately, it had seemed that I was on autopilot. But now there was the promise to be reinvigorated. It was exhilarating and reassuring.

The office is dark and deserted when I return. I head straight for my desk and unlock the cabinet. I lovingly hold my completed application. It's exactly as I left it.

More seriously now, I think again of the yoga training.

Yoga: that tantalizing pipe dream that I'd allowed myself to consider for a few delicious days before smacking myself down for being foolish, and locking the application away. Like Nana's wedding china from 1936, something so precious and fragile that I only took it out of its bubble wrap and used it on the most special of occasions, my imaginary yoga aspirations were a fragile, precious dream that I only dared to examine once in a while. While I worried that Nana's china might break, when it came to my yoga wishes, I worried that if I allowed myself to look too closely, to actually touch this possibility, it might evaporate—*poof*—like the figment of my imagination that it was. And without this dream, without this fantasy of escape, under the weight of the life I'd created for myself, *I* might break.

I should enroll in the yoga training now! I think daringly.

And it really *felt* daring to think these big thoughts and to allow myself the possibility of pursuing this because ordinarily I never look ahead and I seldom look back. I simply do what needs to be done each day, one foot in front of the other, one business trip or project or press conference after the next. Which basically means I subsist on the professional equivalent of gruel—it keeps me alive, but not nourished in any meaningful way. Now, however, raw, tired, and ground down, I let myself think of it. Just a little.

Of course it doesn't mean I'm going to become a yoga teacher, I reason cautiously, in the way that you'll say anything, even if it's not the whole truth, when you're really, really desperate to get something you need. The training itself would be something of substance to look forward to once a month as I continue to work at this job, something to combat the stress. What could be more relaxing than escaping to a beautiful, Zen oasis for a soothing week of yoga this summer, followed by monthly weekend workshops! It would be time set aside for unwinding and recharging, not to mention something that I actually *loved.*

I think of the elegant studio I'd just come from. The dark wood, ornate tapestry, graceful Buddha seated regally at the front...the candlelit class itself. I'd left feeling pampered, utterly relaxed, and recharged. I hadn't wanted to leave at all.

My pulse picks up at the possibility of immersing myself in this serene world. I think of Sweet Pauley. Essentially, here was a way to carve out some space in my life for one thing I *want* to do. And when do we, modern folk with bills to pay, jobs to work, and errands to run, ever stop and think about what we *want*. What we *really, really* want. In a life crowded with things I "have" to do, this would be one precious little nook of freedom and choice. Once a month, I could do yoga all weekend, improve my practice, and head back to work on Monday relaxed and refreshed for the week ahead.

I take a deep, full breath. I can hardly believe this might really happen—that finally, after years of *thinking* about doing something, I'm really *doing* something. I'm applying to yoga training!

I review the application one final time, then fold it ever-so-carefully, place it in an envelope, and drop it into the mailbox on my way home. I stand and listen to the squeaky hinge of the mailbox swallow it irrevocably. It's official: the process is underway.

After three weeks, I still haven't heard back from Thea. Taking my fragile courage in my hands—it's somehow so much harder to be brave when you really care about something—I email to follow up and she immediately responds:

> Hi Sara,
> That's funny. I thought I had already let you know that you're accepted. I think it will be a great fit.
> Many blessings.
> Thea

I've been sitting on the edge of my seat for weeks and she thought she'd already told me? I mentally splutter over this before chalking it up to adorable yogi absentmindedness. *How can she be constrained by day-to-day things like email? She's a real-live yogi, for Pete's sake!*

The important thing is: I'm accepted! I'm going to yoga training!

I think longingly of the beautiful room and Thea's class in candlelight, of the soul-deep sense of peace that soaked into every fiber of my being. I sigh. I want to dive into that world and anoint myself in that yoga peace.

Most of all, I want it to counterbalance the mental fuckery of my corporate life.

Part Two:

From the Conference Room to the Yoga

Mat, Teacher Training Begins

Chapter Seven
Fasten Your Karmic Seat Belt...

...Unexpected Turbulence May Occur

The training begins with a weeklong immersion for which I'd had to withdraw a week's worth of my precious, hard-earned vacation days from the Investorcap bank. This was major. I hoarded those days like a Dickensian miser. And in keeping with the miser theme, I never actually ended up spending them, I just liked knowing they were there for the imaginary aspirational life in which I took fabulous vacations to exotic locations. In reality, I haven't taken a vacation in years. I keep promising myself I will...as soon as I get promoted/finish this project/work slows down/it's summer/it's winter/I can. But I never actually do. Now, however, I'm changing that.

I wake up early on the first day, long before my alarm goes off. Note: this never happens on workdays. I head to the coffee shop on my block since I won't have access to my beloved Keurig machine at work. I feel guilty I haven't gone "drug-free" (caffeine counts by the highest yogic standards) as I'd intended, but I shrug it off. Work has been far too stressful to even consider being as sluggish as I'd be without some coffee. I need to zoom through each day, kicking ass, ticking items off endless lists like a madwoman, and effectively cramming 18 hours of work into ten. After all, that is what's enabled me to do this training.

I savor each sip of my French roast and carefully analyze my yoga wardrobe. I choose my new black pants and gray top featuring a colorful lotus that Nunnally got me in support of my upcoming yoga pursuits. The pants are conservative, classic, and flattering—the yoga equivalent of the little black dress. The shirt has a lotus. What could be more yoga than that?

I pack lunch, vegetarian at least, and tuck the card Nunnally had given me with the new outfit in as a lucky charm. Lunch is always such a social dilemma. As I drive, I worry briefly about who I'll eat with in this new world. But on the positive side, at least I won't have to dodge Vicky and whatever list of imagined transgressions she might have today. I merge onto 93 North, quickly leaving Boston behind. An hour later, I reach the remote outpost in southern New Hampshire where I'll study for the next year. Initially, I'd been disappointed to learn that the trainings weren't held at the luxe Boston studio where Thea teaches, but then became hopeful the training digs would be even more relaxing, in what I imaged would be an idyllic pastoral sanctuary conducive to yoga and creating quiet within.

And although I am officially in the middle of nowhere, this modest, unremarkable, one-story building in a strip mall could hardly be called *idyllic*. Its neighbors are a mini-mart, a chain coffee shop, and a pizza and sandwich joint.

I tell myself not to judge outer appearances. Clearly, what matters is what's within. Feeling smugly yoga-ish, I walk through the glass office door. And stop short. I'd expected to step from the ordinary into Zen—from the strip mall into a spiritual oasis with beautiful wood floors and traditional Indian artwork. I'm woefully disappointed. This is pretty much the opposite of a yogic sanctuary. There are no dancing Bodhisattvas perched intermittently with serene Buddhas. There is no trickling waterfall, no *Sounds of Nature* CD set on loop, no smiling, graceful attendant offering *ayurvedically* balancing tea.

Instead, there's a dull gray carpet and an unattended utilitarian metal desk flanked by two straight-back chairs. It reminds me of the waiting room at the Department of Motor Vehicles.

Ignoring the fact that, like most people, I hate going to the Department of Motor Vehicles, I press on, walking past several empty studios. I easily identify the teacher training room by the long line of Birkenstocks, Crocs, and alterna-hippie footwear yoga practitioners seem to love. I step out of my utterly normal flip-flops and enter the studio.

Again, the anticipated yogic oasis evades me. The requisite stacks of bolsters and blankets are in heaps off to one side, but there the yoga ends. The blankets have only one trait in common and that is that they're all stained and, I find as I approach, somewhat stinky. They aren't the industry-standard traditional Mexican blankets—though why, as an aside, is it industry standard to use blankets from Mexico when the birthland of yoga is India, which is approximately *nowhere near* Mexico?

Ethnic origins of the blankets aside, this studio apparently only provides moving blankets—those that moving companies rent to wrap around your furniture to suggest an air of protection, but in spite of which let your furniture get damaged. Judging from their dingy look and unpleasant odor, these are well used and have never been introduced to a washing machine.

The first one I pick up has been stained by a menstruating prior user. *Eww.* I can't drop it fast enough. A petite blue-eyed blond with white-girl dreadlocks immediately swoops it up and wraps it around herself like a giant, filthy shawl. She drifts away and I sift through the rest of the pile to find one without obvious stains, but even then, I'll cover it with my sweatshirt before settling in. I really want to take a shower in lavender-scented hand sanitizer, but I'll settle for covering it.

The ceilings are low; the lights cold and fluorescent. There is only one window in the long narrow room and light barely penetrates the drawn blinds keeping out pedestrian stares. The group is entirely female and everyone is camped out on the floor—propped up in various poses by a variety of bolsters and moving blankets.

In addition to the blue-eyed blond, some others have actually wrapped these rags around themselves. Yes, it is over-air-conditioned in here, but I would have to be naked, utterly exposed to the elements in the middle of winter, and slathered in a protective layer of hand sanitizer to even *consider* wrapping myself up in any of these.

The class varies widely in age and fitness level. There are only three women you'd look at and think, "Ah yes, she must do yoga."

The one commonality is a nearly across-the-board disregard for personal appearance and in some cases hygiene. Many legs and armpits are unshaven; toenails are unpolished; leggings are paint-splattered, tattered, and torn. Bras are purely optional and mostly foregone. Hair is uncombed, often unwashed, and sometimes dreaded, regardless of race. This crowd is a sharp contrast to the Back Bay beauties, and I suddenly realize that there's a great divide between the people who *teach* and *take* yoga classes. It's both disorienting and slightly exciting to be here, a tourist in the teacher world. *Look! Real, authentic yogis!*

Many trainees seem to already know each other and are enmeshed in deep, impenetrable conversations. A few are reading various interpretations of the *Yoga Sutras* or the *Baghavad Gita*. One woman is sitting in lotus and chanting to herself.

New-girl nerves set in as I search for a good place to sit. It's been 12 years since I've had a first day of school, almost two years since I started at a new job, and seven years since I moved to a new city. I'd allowed myself to find comfort in familiarity. I'd forgotten how scary change can be, and how alone and unsure one can feel.

I see a Hispanic woman with a friendly smile and sit down next to her, introducing myself. Noemi tells me she commutes from Chicago.

The idea of someone commuting from Chicago is so outlandish that I almost ask, "Is that north of here?" as though it's just another New England town before I realize she means *Chicago*, as in the one in Illinois.

I shake her hand and lead with what I know best: food. "Welcome to New England! Let me know if you need any restaurant recommendations. I love to eat."

Then I notice her shirt. In bold, graphic letters, stretched across her braless chest, is the incontrovertible word "VAGINA!" Unsure of what to do—stare? ask? nod approvingly?—I try to ignore it. She tells me she works as a psychologist with immigrant families. She seems friendly, open, and sweet. Tiny miniature car earrings dangle from each ear. She appeals to my secret alterna-funky side—the part of me that I carefully hide from my corporate colleagues. The part that yearns to skip wearing a bra for once in my life—or at least skip wearing suits—and maybe, just maybe, one day even wear a T-shirt that shamelessly shouts, "Vagina!"

Then again...do I really need to announce my genitals on a T-shirt? Does anyone? I wouldn't think a "penis" T-shirt was cool. And really, if you start there, where do you stop? "Labia"? "Testicles"? Or the gender-neutral, "Anus"? Does anyone actually need an "Anus" shirt?

Unfortunately, I can think of several who do.

As this is yoga teacher training, and because everyone else is doing it and I'm not immune to peer pressure, I feel the need to attempt lotus, even though my knees strain to get there and my chronically tight hips never let it feel comfortable. After I wind my legs as close to the pose as they're going to get, I look around at my fellow trainees. To my surprise, the entire room is women, about 20 in all. There is not a single male in sight. Sure, I'd vaguely noticed over the years that most teachers were women. But because the classes were always coed, it had never really stuck out. Now, however, the sheer overwhelming femaleness of the room is startling.

It's diametrically opposite from life at the office. I'm used to being the token woman there, engulfed by my male colleagues and their talk of sports, chicks, and carousing. In an effort to blend in, my first task Monday mornings is to check all the local teams' scores so I can keep up on one front at least. Unless I'm with the admins, I carefully conceal all traces of female interests. Melding myself into the male corporate culture is a sacrifice I willingly make to fit in. Here, on the other hand, it's clear that my gender won't be an obstacle to my cultural integration. If anything, I suspect it will be my corporateness; my commitment to personal hygiene; and my utter lack of piercings, tattoos, and swirly, stained, gypsy clothes.

I turn to my other side as a pale woman who fits right in with paisley pants and a medley of assorted colors on top, starts setting up camp—a full arsenal of blankets, bolsters, and blocks—far too close to me. I look around at the respectable, normal distance between each yogini in the rest of the circle, and then at my new neighbor, whose blanket is now touching mine. Apologetically, I inch away to give us both some room.

"I'm Gloria," she says, twined into lotus in the middle of her campsite, looking up with an eager intractability I'd never heard in anyone before. Her light brown hair is wound into a single side braid. "But I'm thinking of taking a yoga name like Prana...or maybe Bhakti. I'm a freecyclables artist—you know, I go through other people's trash and make art out of their discarded objects. But I only work when I'm inspired…when my creativity is ready to be expressed as tangible works."

"Hi, I'm Sara—" I begin, but Gloria/Prana-Bhakti cuts in. "Have you ever considered taking a yoga name?"

"Uh, no, I haven't yet." Never have and never will, would be more accurate. "I think I'll just stay…you know, Sara."

There's a long pause as she looks disappointed at my lack of interest in a yoga name (whatever that is). I briefly imagine her retelling her yoga friends, "This poor corporate soul…she's just not *ready*." She yanks me back to the present moment by telling me that her son is 98 months and 11 days old.

I try to take that in stride, "Oh, wow. That's interesting…why…um…do you measure in months and days?"

"Life is too precious to waste even a day lumping things into years," she answers in her eager way, smiling, waiting for me to agree with her.

I wonder how old I am in months, try to do the math, and give up.

I look up as the blue-eyed blond in my discarded blanket walks over. I'm relieved at the potential exit from my strange conversation with Gloria/Prana-Bhakti.

"I *knew* something made me stop here," she says. Half-standing, she gives me a hug—which means that she sort of hugs my head while my face is squashed into her cleavage. Mid-hug, I feel her smelling my neck. "Wow! White people really do smell like milk!"

The fact that she herself is white seems to be lost on her. She sinks down in front of me and settles into lotus with our knees touching. Around us, there's the overwhelming smell of sweaty feet and unwashed bodies. "I'm Summer," she tells me. She goes on to say she's on an "indefinite break" from studying music, and specifically percussion, at college. She doesn't shave or wear a bra. Everything she's wearing appears to be torn or paint-splattered. Her youth-sized peace-sign shirt— both torn *and* paint-splattered—is layered on top of an orange top. Layering seems to be big in the yoga world.

"I'm into growing my own herbs and roots," she tells me when I ask what she's doing on her indefinite college break. She goes on to say she uses her herbs and roots for brewing tea and "healing things," and, in fact, grew the roots that brewed the tea she's currently drinking.

"Sip?" she offers with a wide, sweet smile, holding out a recycled jelly jar full of muddy-looking liquid. I'm flattered at her generous offer to share her brew, but horrified by the potential germ-sharing with a total stranger, especially one who doesn't share my disdain for the stained blankets.

She keeps smiling and beaming out the friendship vibe even after I politely decline the concoction. She seems totally guileless. I bet she's a youngest child…or maybe high. I feel the need to take care of her.

The door opens and heads whip expectantly, then turn back, disappointed, when it's not Thea. Instead, a beautiful Mediterranean-looking woman with long jet-black hair hurries in and claims the last open space in the circle, closest to the door. She's wearing a vibrant pink, silky dress. It makes a dramatic contrast to the attire of the rest of the class, who not only don't seem to have given a single thought to their appearance, but are actually throwing out the vibe that they're oh-so-much-more-yogic *because* of their renunciation of material goods.

"I've heard Thea described as both a demon and a goddess," Summer whispers. "I wonder which it is."

The door opens again. This time chatter ceases, replaced by an awed silence that washes over the room; Thea, tiny, brawny pixie that she is, has arrived.

There is something truly intimidating about her—not just because she has a doctorate and tours internationally, not just because she has her own teacher-training program, not just because she is a bit of a local celebrity, and not because, as demonstrated on her website, she can do incredible arm balances. No, Thea's intimidating because everything about her from her stance to her comments, to her energy, makes it clear that she has very definitive boundaries and you aren't welcome inside them.

After a cursory greeting of hands in prayer and head bowed—and reciprocal responses from the students—Thea begins, "Yoginis, *namaste*. Before we start, we should talk about the importance of boundaries. Now, what do I mean by that?"

Almost every hand in the room rams up at dizzying speed. Thea nods permission to speak toward a pale woman who looks like she did her hair with a bucket of mousse and a top-down convertible. The short, light brown strands stick straight out of her scalp in every direction. I decide her yoga name would be Disheveled Yoga Hair.

Wearing a grand hodgepodge of way too many bright colors, the woman clasps her hands at her heart and nod-bows in return. "Do you mean providing limits for ourselves in order to protect our energetic supply in the psychic realm and the safety of our physical bodies?"

"Hmm. That's part of it," Thea says while I wonder what the heck that means. "But I also want to talk about the importance of boundaries between teacher and students. I often have students come up to talk to me at the grocery store and look into my cart, asking what I eat and how I stay so thin. And recently I was almost mobbed at a national conference. I had to wear giant, movie star sunglasses and my assistants had to act as bodyguards, keeping the crowds back just so I could get from one place to another—from my lecture to lunch. I was even followed into the pool when I went for a swim! People kept wanting to know everything about me...my diet, exercise, personal life...."

Disheveled Yoga Hair shakes her head sadly. "As though you would ever be concerned with such *prakriti*—that means the physical body of this lifetime," she translates for the rest of us.

Ignoring her, I wonder who the brave souls (or oblivious idiots) are who would dare to approach Thea in public, let alone mob her at a national conference. Are they completely insane? Immune from the laws of psychics in the natural world?

"And you wouldn't believe the emails I get!" Thea holds up a stack of emails from people as far away as Australia writing to her about their asphyxiating anxiety, their devastating depression, their innumerable physical ailments. She reads one from a student who recently moved to the area and, thinking Thea had seemed cool, had asked her for bar recommendations.

There is a collective, condemning gasp. "Bars?! You mean…for drinking?"

"Yeah, that's *real* yogic. She probably does power yoga too," Disheveled Yoga Hair scoffs indignantly.

In this Puritanical kingdom, the idea that someone would ask Thea, the grand yoga pooh-bah, for recommendations on where to partake of forbidden drink is nothing less than scandalous. I redden guiltily. I should've pushed myself harder on the whole yogic sobriety thing. I don't dare mention my start in power yoga.

"Yogis, we have to remember to lend others our light," Thea says, stemming the tide of criticism.

Immediately, there's a swift reversal in comments.

"Absolutely, Thea. We need to maintain compassion," Disheveled Yoga Hair says authoritatively.

"Maybe she'll get there someday…you know, *in her own time*.…"

"Oh *of course*…yoga is there for everyone…when she's ready to see the path, it will appear. Not everyone's ready to do the work and self-study to be a yogi right now."

"Yes, that's true," Thea agrees, "but I was sharing this more as an example of how we have to be really careful about our boundaries."

"Guys, Thea's raising a really valid point. We need to be careful with our boundaries," Disheveled Yoga Hair says.

"Yeah, boundaries are *so* important," a tall, skinny blond agrees.

Thea nods, then continues to talk about violations of her boundaries. As she does, she might as well be erecting an electric fence around herself. There is her…and then there are the marauding invaders of her privacy. She makes it clear you don't want to be one of them. The more she speaks disdainfully about this, the more certain I am that I will never dare to ask her any questions or even approach her outside of this training. If I ever have the stupendous misfortune of accidentally running into her while grocery shopping, I will avoid eye contact at all costs. I'd sooner stab myself with toothpicks than look in her cart or ask what she eats, sooner starve than ask for a restaurant recommendation, sooner sizzle to a sunburned crisp than take a dip in the same pool. If anything, I will be the student she thinks of fondly who she never really knew.

Invisible fence fully operational, she reaches into a huge box of photocopies and starts passing them out in five-inch stacks to each of the 22 trainees now sitting in the ragged circle.

"I must owe a karmic debt to the copy place," she says and everyone giggles readily. "And whatever it is, it must've been something really bad"—this is greeted with more giggles at the incongruity that Thea could ever do something bad, let alone *really* bad—"because that place manages to mess up all my orders. So we're going to have to sort and collate these ourselves."

I stare at the 500 to 600 pages of copies in front of me dubiously. *We actually have to organize these huge stacks?* Then: *Wait, we actually have to* read *these stacks?* I guess I hadn't thought about what sort of reading would be required for yoga teacher training. But I surely hadn't anticipated *this*.

The next half-hour is spent asking which pages people have, which they need, and putting them in some sort of order. I note that organization is not a key strength of most of these yogis, as cries of, "Wait, *which* one goes next?" lengthen the process. My inner obsessive-compulsive screams for release.

When everyone's as organized as they're going to get, which is about as organized as a roomful of two-year olds hyped up on espresso and surrounded by puppies, Thea announces we will break into pairs with the yogi next to us, chat for a minute, and introduce each other to the group. Paired with Gloria (I mentally drop the Prana-Bhakti from her name), I learn she lives in Portsmouth, a charming town on the coast of New Hampshire, with her husband, who she refers to as her "partner," and son. I give her the barebones facts about me: I live in Boston, work in financial services, and am engaged. I casually mention that Nunnally grew up in Portsmouth. "Small world," I add with a smile.

"This is Gloria," I say in my professional presenting voice when it's my turn. "She lives in Portsmouth with her husband and son." I leave out the possible yoga name change, the partner-husband thing, and the month age-counting.

When it's time to return the favor, Gloria takes a different approach. "And this is the very lovely *Sara*." She lingers over the last two syllables and I can tell she's still thinking about a future yoga moniker for me. "She was drawn here because her spirit is yearning for a yogic oasis...."

Wait...what? I feel myself start blushing.

"...She is pledged to her soul partner...."

Pledged? Soul partner?

"...Our paths have already crossed—karma, destiny—as he apparently grew up in the town where I currently call my home...well, you know, my material, physical home...for this moment...in this lifetime at least."

My brain involuntarily wonders where her non-physical home is.

"...*Sara* is here to—"

I'm waiting for it. Scared, but waiting.

She gestures circularly with her hands, "—evolve," hand twirl, hand twirl. "Explore yoga. Be yoga. Isn't that lovely? Yoga as life. *Namaste*." The hand-twirling concludes with a swirl that ends in prayer hands over her heart. She bows her head over them.

She leans in after the announcement and whispers, "Sorry— I get word vomit. You know, where you can't stop talking? It's like diarrhea, but vomit? You know?"

Smiling carefully, I turn away, fervently hoping that will cure all vomiting (and any diarrhea). "I'm just here to learn as much as I can." I add aloud to the group in a "nothing more to see here, folks; move along now" tone, hoping I seem likable and normal. Mentally, I add, *I'm also here to get away from my job and get better at yoga, and if, in the process, my arms accidentally get more toned for the wedding, so be it.*

The introductions snake around the circle. There are a few graduate students who are finishing their degrees in psychology or social work, a part-time bodyworker, a professional ballerina, some full-time moms, a retired grade-school teacher, some yoga teachers, a handful of unemployed soul-searchers, and Gloria, the freecyclables artist. I'm the only one with a full-time corporate job. The only one who works the Monday to Friday, eight-to-five schedule by which I thought *everyone* lived.

Thea suggests we commence our year of training with an opening chant to bless the guru-student relationship, our learning, and our interactions.

Wait—what? Up to this point, nothing has been what I expected. I feel alone and out of place. In terms of the location or the interactions, it's certainly not the Zen paradise I was expecting. And now...blessing our interactions? Sure, I figured I'd have to join in on an "OM" or two when we did yoga, but anything beyond that is weird. The Tri Dosha Yoga website hadn't said anything about this. The more-straitlaced side of my inner duality rears back. I've never chanted in my life. The closest thing in my experience is that I once *heard* a Gregorian monk CD at a spa where I'd gotten a detoxifying facial—and I certainly hadn't joined in.

My lifelong fear of singing in public immediately rises up in front of me. I blush as I anticipate condemning gazes shifting toward me, the horrendous singer. Thankfully, everyone else's eyes are closed as Thea leads some sort of "centering meditation," about allowing ourselves to evolve.

I snap my eyes shut in an effort to get with the program. This valiant attempt lasts about two seconds. I can't stop wondering what I'm missing. So I peek and see, again, that everyone else still has their eyes closed—which makes me feel even weirder, like when you're in the midst of passionate kissing, but then you peek at the other person only to see that he's not, and then you feel guilty and weird and totally out of the moment.

I firmly resolve to focus and chant. *I'm here for new experiences. If chanting is called for, chant I shall.* Thea leads off, in Sanskrit apparently, and everyone else seems to know that this will be a call-and-response situation. Aside from a few pose names, I've never heard this language before. Endless jumbles of syllables whiz past; I can't latch on to any.

All around, it sounds like a loudest-chanter competition. But I shrink into my own silence. I try to picture telling my coworkers that I took a week off work and paid thousands of dollars to…*chant*. I imagine the bemused looks I'd get in return, and know that I never will reveal this at the office, or, frankly, anywhere outside this room.

Silence stretches after the chant.

Finally, Thea speaks. "In addition to this weeklong immersion, we require you to attend monthly workshops; complete self-study and homework questions, which are due seven days after the workshops; take a minimum of one regular yoga class with me per month; and complete 40 hours assisting my classes under my supervision. Assisting is really important—you need to have a full repertoire of adjustments at your disposal. You'll also need to have a strong grasp of Sanskrit, the language of yoga, and be fluent in all the pose names. Lastly, you'll also be required to complete both individual and group projects."

Already familiar with these requirements from my original research, I nonetheless take careful notes in my plain, spiral-bound notebook. Everyone, looking as though this is brand new information, scribbles excitedly in their embroidered, yoga-themed journals.

Thea goes on to explain that unlike other training programs that require you to complete 200 hours of training in order to awarded the 200-hour certification, we'll actually undergo 400 hours of training to be awarded the same 200-hour designation.

I raise my chin proudly; I chose the right course. The time, the money, the increased hours…other programs seem so woefully insufficient by comparison.

"At the end of the year, three yoginis will be chosen for yearlong teaching apprenticeships called the *Seva* Rotations, at studios in Boston and New Hampshire that we have partnerships with. But try not to let that distract from your studies. *Seva* translates to selfless service, in Sanskrit. And I've found that this works best when we allow this opportunity to rise organically." She smiles again.

Excitement pulses through the room. For new teachers, the opportunity is high value, providing the "chosen ones" with an introduction to the teaching community and real-world experience in a competitive, saturated market. I feel both left out and proud of the fact that I'm merely here to deepen my studies. At least I don't have to compete for a *Seva* spot.

"Our goal is to enable our students to feel empowered in their own right. As teachers, we should always try to be humble and remember that it's not us—it's the yoga. It's the work that people do themselves and their willingness to let go that determines their transformation," Thea instructs.

Until now, I'd never thought about the possibility of some sort of transformation through yoga. I'd tried yoga in the first place because my heart was broken and I'd needed to pour myself into something. I'd stayed because it made me feel physically strong and mentally calm. Since I'd started taking Thea's classes, I'd also noted a spiritual element—alone a mental leap for me. If I'd thought about it any further, and, frankly, I hadn't, I would've assumed that physical exhaustion begot mental peace. But it seemed that Thea was talking about something much more than that. Which made me wonder: Does that transformation happen by itself or do you actually have to do something to accomplish it?

"As the schedule indicates, starting tomorrow, we'll begin our days with anatomy and spend afternoons on yoga theory. For today, however, we'll just focus on yoga theory."

With that, we're dismissed for 45 minutes before the afternoon session.

Disheveled Yoga Hair, whose real name, I'd learned during introductions, is Brinley, announces to no one/everyone that her inner essence can only be rebalanced with an inversion and tips up into a headstand. Summer looks around, emitting something between a nervous giggle and a helpless gasp. Gloria begins dramatically sketching on an art pad she whips out of nowhere. A few others flop on their backs wherever they're sitting like felled toy soldiers. But the majority sprint toward Thea and spread out at her feet as though we hadn't talked endlessly about the importance of boundaries and how Thea's constantly fending off adoring fans.

Brinley descends from her headstand in time to saunter over and reclaim her seat. It's approximately four centimeters to Thea's left. "I'd like to talk about yoga and motherhood…ever since my daughter was born, my practice, and my relationship to that practice, has changed."

Avoiding eye contact—*see Thea? I'd never violate your boundaries!*—I rush outside. Despite my fervent desire to sit in the sun, and the fact that I'm a professional woman approaching the age of 30 who should not think twice about it, I'm still ridiculously shy about walking across the street toward a small group from class that is sitting on the grass near some picnic benches. I rein myself in, assuring myself that yogis are renowned for their kindness and acceptance of all. With a deep breath, I make myself go over. "Hi everybody, I'm Sara," I say, still self-conscious, as I sit down and unpack my insulated lunch bag.

The beautiful Mediterranean-looking woman in the pink dress who had hurried in late, reciprocates. "Hi! I'm Jessica, and I guess I'm a sucker for learning because I'm also pursuing my master's in classics full time while I work at a museum downtown."

"Oh cool!" I say. "I love history—in fact, it was my minor."

Her face lights up. "Fellow history geek!"

"And fellow fashion-lover—I have that same dress in black," I tell her. "Isn't it the best? I wear it everywhere from work to travel to parties."

"Totally. I wear it all the time too. *Clearly.*" She laughs again. "I'm the only one who's crazy enough to wear a dress to a yoga thing, but I brought leggings for just such an occasion." She gestures to sitting on the ground.

I'm more impressed that she's in full lotus, each ankle resting on the opposite thigh, knees fully down. I marvel at her ability to sit this way in a dress, on the grass, and yet look completely at home doing so.

I've noticed an interesting phenomenon with women whereby the pretty one is often ostracized, back-stabbed, or ignored. Not me—I want to befriend her. I've never understood the need to push other women down, professionally or personally, pretty or not. Why wouldn't you want to share with, learn from, and help your fellow females? Life is hard enough—we don't need to make it additionally harder on anyone, let alone our own gender.

"It's really pretty," Hazel adds. A photographer around my age with the kind of thick, shiny blond mane I hadn't known existed outside shampoo commercials, Hazel exudes a slow-moving, calm consideration of life as it goes on around her, yet a deep groundedness that prevents her from being disturbed by it in any way. I envy that.

"It reminds me of a dress this woman was wearing for a photo shoot I did last week."

"That's awesome that you're a photographer," I say. "I've always wondered what that would be like."

"Yeah, it's fun," Hazel says, turning left to face Jaznae. "What about you? What do you do for work?"

Jaznae says simply, "I'm an artist." But with her pronunciation, it sounds like, "Ah'm an *ahteest*."

Intrigued by her accent (I can't place it though…something island-y?) and profession, I can barely contain my excitement. "You are? That's *so* cool!" I exclaim, in a manner that's the antithesis of cool. "What's your medium? Watercolor? Oil? Pottery?"

Jaznae does not look up from her food, or miss even a beat of chewing. "It does not matter which." (This sounds like: "Eet does naught matter wheech.") "You only need to know that I'm an ahteest." Her tone implies that only superficial assholes concern themselves with details. She ignores Jessica and Hazel altogether.

I'm embarrassed—as though I got caught asking an inappropriate question like, "How much money do you actually make?" Or to borrow a phrase from my work-buddy Betsy, "How many people have you done the wild honky with?"

I really don't want to get off on the wrong foot with any of my classmates, especially on the first day. We'll be spending the next year together. I quickly backpedal. "I was just asking because I think it's really cool," I explain hastily. "Art's so cool! I'd love to hear all about it." *Stop talking. Stop saying "cool,"* I tell myself, wondering if Gloria's word-vomit is contagious.

Jaznae doesn't bother to look at me, still focused on chewing, looking down at her lunch. "I don't define myself by what I do. I'm an ahteest. That is my inner essence. That is all you need to know. My urban shaman is defined by her shaman inner essence. Yes, she also cleans toilets. But really, she is an urban shaman." Her icy tone indicates that the conversation is now over.

Jessica rolls her eyes. Hazel keeps calmly eating her salad.

"Well I don't define myself by what I do either. But we were just talking about what we do, not inner essences," I say, mentally *adding whatever those are.*

"I do not weigh myself down like that. I'm spiritually *free*," Jaznae says.

I have no response for that. We finish eating in silence.

Heading back inside, I'm careful to avoid the cluster around Thea as I reluctantly return to my spot. Jessica does the same. Apparently, however, not everyone is of the same mindset. Presumably having foregone their lunch break, the same group is still clamoring around Thea. They wilt with disappointment as she stands and announces that she needs to refresh her herbal tea. There is a flurry of offers to do this for her, which she refuses. As she heads out, there is a subsequent flurry of offers to go with her, which she also firmly shoots down, but some still straggle after her, claiming to coincidentally need tea themselves. The rest of the group disperses, the air heavy with disappointment.

Disbanded from the Thea hoverers, Summer sits down next to my feet. She smiles dreamily and pulls a head of purple cabbage out of her yoga bag. She peels the layers off one by one and eats them. Raw and plain.

Harper, a grad student from Tennessee, reaches for some sort of shepherd's cane device that she proceeds to hook over her shoulder and massage herself with vigorously. Then she passes it around the circle. Yogi by yogi, the self-massaging commences. Eager to be part of the group, I accept my turn, hooking it into my back and wiggling it around, hoping that's how it's actually done. And even though it's weird, I'm grateful to work on the knots in my back from sitting on the floor all day.

After a few minutes, Thea returns (with a few tea drinkers in tow) for three hours of lecture on yoga.

"Let's discuss the difference between a good class and a transformational experience. A good class can be technically sound and injury-free. And that's a valid experience...." She pauses long enough to imply, *if you're satisfied with run-of-the-mill crap.* "But a *transformational* teacher who transcends the boundaries of *asana* and physical practice to an experience that truly provides students with the opportunity for something beyond...well, that transcendence has nothing to do with your knowledge of anatomy and everything to do with the essential guidance and care you extend to your students. That's the inner essence of a transformational teacher."

It sounds so beautiful, so yogic. I wish I could think of things like that. But embarrassingly, I still don't really understand the concept of "inner essence," let alone the rest. Maybe it's a yoga-thing.

"As you teach, you lend your students your light and compassion as a lamp to guide them through the maze of their inner selves. As you unwind the emotional and mental tangles they hold in the mental, emotional, and physical realms—and the ramifications of those tangles, a lot of issues can come up for both you, as a teacher, as well as them, as students. This can take the form of transference and countertransference within your interactions."

Everyone nods as though that makes perfect sense. I succumb to herd mentality and do the same even though I really have no idea what she is talking about.

While everyone else continues nodding, I start to feel a tendril of anxiety. I didn't think I'd be delving into this sort of psychology stuff. Foolishly, I thought I'd actually be doing yoga. I imagine raising my hand and asking if I've mistakenly come to a support group instead. *Um...I'm here for the yoga? Yoga, anyone, yoga?*

The key, Thea explains, is to use a technique of focused observation, compassionate acknowledgment, and nonattached validation. "You know how chefs wear kitchen whites to keep them safe from splatters and burns? Well, we'll be working on building our yoga whites—the barriers that will keep you safe from emotional splatters and burns." She smiles delightedly and sips her herbal tea.

But can't I just do yoga instead and avoid all burns? Can't we work on alignment and learn how to do cool arm balances?

"Know your own limits," Thea advises. "There will be issues in our lives that affect us and our teaching. The key is compartmentalizing, being able to ritualize the passage from one container into another with strong boundaries between each."

In this already long day of indecipherable psychologisms, the last incomprehensible one renders me most dumbstruck. But once again, everyone is nodding thoughtfully, as though talk of "ritualized passage" and "containers" is completely normal. Surely, I cannot be the only one who thinks of containers as Tupperware. But judging from all the nodding, you'd think I *was* the only one.

Sudden terrifying thought: *maybe I really* am *the only one.* I nod my head anyway.

"Let's explore how we practice our emotional self-care rituals," Thea says, launching into a discussion of how some people recharge themselves emotionally.

Despite the weird New-Age-y-ness of this (is everything a practice or a ritual around here?), I consider what my "self-care ritual" is, and it is…nonexistent. I only recharge when I'm so worn down, worn thin, and worn out that I completely hit a wall. Then I take a day or two off from my soul-sucking, life-draining job, stay home, take hot bubble baths, gobble vitamins, and sleep a lot. Next, I return to work, wash, rinse, and repeat. But what would my life be like if I didn't wait until I hit that wall? What if I learned and implemented this whole "self-care" concept—which to be honest, still strikes me as perilously New-Age-y and best intoned breathily from within a haze of incense? I *so* do not want to be one of those people going around saying, "Sorry, I can't meet you Friday. I'm having a self-care night," *à la* one of those people everyone dreads who goes around saying, "My therapist says…." But seriously, what if this self-care thing really did become part of my routine life instead of an emergency measure?

What if I learned the concept of self-care instead of wearing my non-care like a badge of pride. Maybe self-care's not just for sissies and the chronically self-indulgent. My mother was a notorious self-care-neglector and was diagnosed with terminal breast cancer at the age of 49.

Brinley's hand rams up. "I'd like to share *my* self-care with the group," she says.

Thea nods her permission.

Brinley closes her eyes and takes her time to shift and readjust herself. Slowly, she clears her throat. "Self-care has become even more important to me since The Birth." The way she articulates it, *The Birth* is definitely capitalized to convey its great import.

"When my daughter was born, she became my whole life and taking care of her, being there for her, and fulfilling my role as a mother were the only things that mattered. But my self-care suffered." Her voice trails off and she looks crestfallen, yet still meditative. "And *now* self-care has to become an even bigger ritual I need to incorporate into my life. My baby, Persephone, is my entire life. But my life is also yoga, yoga is my life. Self-care is yoga. Yoga is self-care." The wisdom-sharing complete, she smiles beatifically at the circle, brings her palms together at her heart, and bows her head over them.

Thea is smiling and nodding. "Good. It's almost time to wrap up for the day. I know this was a lot, and we moved around a bit, but one of the most important things to remember as you undertake this transformational year is not to get too worried about structure. Just allow yourself to receive all that we're covering on some very primal level."

That sounds very yogic, and is meant to be reassuring. However, it only manages to unnerve me further. I thrive on structure. I love structure. I insert structure wherever and whenever I can—home, work, gym, yoga, friendships, and relationships. "What can I say? I like to be organized," I once told my friend Leigh after a deeply satisfying cleaning rampage she assisted me with.

"One might say even *obsessively* organized," she'd clarified kindly, with only the tiniest bit of irony as she printed labels on her label maker and handed me a "Misc."

Without regard for my angst, Thea presses on. "In addition, I want you to keep in mind that painful experiences present chances for growth. Next time you encounter pain, resistance, or emotional discomfort, allow yourself to feel the suffering and reach a deeper understanding, rather than just finding the fastest way possible to stop feeling the pain. Don't just reach for the emotional aspirin. Sit and feel what you're feeling."

I shift nervously on my bolster. I'd actually prefer to avoid pain if at all possible. Given the apparent nature of this training and the intensity of my fellow trainees, some sort of painful initiation by means of bodily or mental pain certainly doesn't seem out of the realm of possibilities. I want to ask if there is any other form of torture available as a substitute. *Hard work? Studying? An extra project, perhaps?*

Predictably, Brinley raises her hand. "I'd like to offer the group an example from my own life," she says in her slow, deliberate way, brow furrowed with concentration. The purposefulness of her words reminds me of a show I'd once seen on the History Channel depicting sages being spoken to from the great beyond.

"I've had a wandering spleen for most of my life. Especially since The Birth of my daughter, and now with carrying her around all the time"—she mimes rocking a baby in her arms—"it all puts extra strain on my trunk. For a long time, I suffered with this pain, and my suffering was just that...*pain*. But now in my work as a yoga therapist intern, I use my knowledge of that pain to better understand and empathize with my clients. It's been an *opportunity*."

Thea rewards her with a nod. "Great example, Brinley."

Brinley smiles proudly.

"Transformation and transcendence:" Thea says, "to bring growth to that which is dormant. This training is a chance for you to burn off the outer layers of your material existence and let the nucleus of your being move toward the ultimate liberation of spiritual transcendence without the painful experiences that usually precede growth."

She pauses. I try to absorb that and immediately fail. I'm too busy thinking about the fact that this is only day one.

Thea ends the day with another group chant.

I think of the mountain of information I just digested—or didn't digest, as the case may be. *Holy. Freaking. Crap.* I feel like I've fallen through a hole in the space-time continuum and into an alternate universe whose language and ways are completely foreign to me. Panic looms.

Chapter Eight
Krishna, You Know It Ain't Easy

To Wax and to Wane

By the fifth day of our training, it feels like a time warp. It's possible we've been here for years. It certainly *seems* like years. We begin each morning with our anatomy teacher, a woman named Ronnie, who is a professor of physical therapy at a local university. And despite spending hours each day immersed in "the language of the body," I can say with certainty that anatomy, much like chanting in Sanskrit, is yet another foreign language.

"Anterior, posterior, medial, lateral, superficial, deep...the saggital plane, the coronal plane, the transverse plane...206 bones...639 muscles...axial... appendicular... protracting, retracting...lateral mediation...." For long stretches, the lectures sound like the adults in a Peanuts cartoon, *"Wah, wah, wah, wah, wah, wah, wahhhhh."*

Out of the blue, Brinley raises her hand and blurts out, "When are we going to cover ligaments? Specifically, the weakening of ligaments and how that might affect someone's practice? I ask because of my wandering spleen and I want to make sure we spend enough time on it—both the emotional and physical aspects. But I'm willing to address the emotional later in Thea's part."

I glance over at Jessica, and she rolls her eyes knowingly. Jessica is one of those people who you click with and then feel like you've known for years, which has been key to survival in this parallel yoga universe. Both the overwhelming flow of foreign information that comprises each day and the overwhelming sensitivity and oddities of some of the trainees with whom we share each day have made that survival equally challenging. So far, Brinley has managed to conspicuously reference her wandering spleen at least once per session. I stare at her purple headband, wondering if she thinks it somehow coordinates with her florescent tie-dyed leggings and orange and lime shirt. She is a riot of wild colors.

"That's an exceedingly rare condition, Brinley, and we won't be able to specifically cover it today, but I'd be happy to discuss with you at another time," Ronnie says firmly.

Scolded, Brinley retreats, visibly sulking.

Ronnie returns to her lecture, and, as per usual, I take notes as fast as my cramping hand, used to typing on a keyboard and unused to clenching a pen, will go. In what can only be described as anatomy waterboarding, Ronnie inundates us with information and I try desperately to swoop up as much as possible in my butterfly net brain, but the net seems to have holes the size of Montana, and I can't seem to grasp anything. Prior to today, the closest I'd gotten to anatomy and physiology was scoping the Friday night bar scene with Leigh back in our single days.

Ronnie flips to a new chart. "Blood production happens in the bones. The ones that don't produce blood are just filled with fat. When you cut into them, they're blubbery yellow. You know, like when you cut into a chicken bone, and sometimes it's yellow, sometimes it's red."

There is a collective look of disgust and a resounding "*ewwww.*" Brinley makes a show of gagging. She looks like she might actually vomit. Maybe right here and now.

Instead, she raises her hand, looking very righteous. "*Ronnie,* could we find a more mindful example in line with the yogic values of *ahimsa*, nonviolence? *Most* of us—if not *all* of us—" she sends a sweeping accusatory glare around the room "—are practicing *ahimsa* through vegetarianism."

"Sorry, vegetarians," Ronnie says to the room in general, not sounding sorry at all. "We're meat. They're meat. A tofu comparison just won't work."

Ronnie goes on to list the five other types of synovial joints and examples of each, but my brain is on one last tic of battery and I zone out. My back aches from sitting on the floor and I'm now officially on overload. Ordinarily intrigued by both new information and foreign languages, today I can't seem to understand anything. Obviously, in Latin, the language of anatomy, I'm a *stupida assinus*.

As Ronnie moves on to the biomechanical details of healthy knee function, I glance around at the group. Over the past week, I've done one-on-one partner work with both Jessica and Hazel, as well as with Kim, an outgoing blond psychologist around my age, and Janet, a retired grade-school teacher with long salt-and-pepper dreadlocks, deep brown skin the color of milk chocolate, and a ready smile. In combination, this small group has come to form a shelter from the larger group.

Our training days have taken on a well-oiled mechanical rhythm. Mornings begin with Ronnie nearly drowning us with information on things like synovial joints, fascia, and cartilage. Invariably, we're then unwillingly enlightened as to how one issue or another affects Brinley's wandering spleen or The Birth of her daughter. Various other students, terrified to be left out and only too eager to demonstrate their innate yogic understanding of anatomy, then share their own anatomical issues. Then Summer might share how she's creating a drum solo inspired by cartilage and Gloria will alert us as to how this has translated into her freecycle art.

At lunch, Jessica and I go running. Sometimes Summer comes along, braless and barefoot. When she does, she slows down the pace. I try not be annoyed, to remember that I don't have to adhere unbendingly to my usual routines. Everyday doesn't have to be a grinding, unyielding race against time…it just *feels* like it does.

Afternoons are comprised of yoga theory with Thea, who floods us with concepts like rituals, transformation, containers, and boundaries. Invariably, we're then unwillingly enlightened as to how these affect Brinley's wandering spleen and The Birth of her daughter. Others then race to explain what rituals, transformations, and containers mean to them. Summer and Gloria may or may not explain what they're creating inspired by the terms *du jour*. The result of which is the time-warp phenomenon.

Finally, drowning in a sea of information and mentally gasping for air, we are dismissed for the day. I then drive home and stare at the homework, trying not to panic. This is the sequence of our days, every day.

Resolutely, I pull my attention back to Ronnie and the biomechanics of the knee. "Now, let's move on to meniscocapsular aponeurosis...." Hopelessly lost, I write it down.

As soon as we are settled for an afternoon of yoga theory with Thea, Summer immediately raises her hand. "Thea? I really want to experience a spiritual transformation, but it isn't happening."

Thea smiles warmly, seeming to have no particular urgency to answer. She looks at Summer and nods encouragingly.

Silence pervades the big room.

Finally Janet, my retired teacher buddy, speaks up. "Honey, it'll happen when it happens. Don't try to rush your life's events."

"So...just keep waiting?" Summer seems disappointed yet resigned to this.

Everyone nods.

"Ah, to be young and eager," someone says with just enough knowing to sound a trace condescending.

Thea smiles and nods, possibly agreeing, or maybe just for the sake of it. Or to stretch her neck muscles. Or perhaps to maintain strong teacher-student boundaries. A week in this alien world and I can't tell for certain. "Today we're looking at the mind-body connection—as well as the ideas of being able to create and heal various physical and mental issues, the ramifications of sexual repression, shame, guilt, fear, desire, jealousy, hatred, and the complexity of your emotional currency."

Oh goody, an easy day.

Brinley speaks up. "Ever since The Birth, I've tried to be mindful of the challenge of balancing how I relate to myself as a mother and how I relate to myself as a wife and yogi...the relations and grounding of these roles in my life seem correlated to the internal visceral relations of my wandering spleen."

I try to refrain from rolling my eyes. Brinley and her WS have been the class' most constant companions this week. If we were a sports team, our mascot would be her daughter dressed as a wandering spleen. If I never again hear about either, it will be a day too soon.

Thea nods. "The myriad relations that exist within the mind-body realm are undeniable."

I pry my eyeballs back from out of my skull.

The next day, after another overwhelming anatomy lecture, I skip running and head straight toward the picnic benches across the street. Beyond the picnic area, there is a small pond—more of a giant puddle, actually. A giant puddle with an inordinate number of ducks. There are "no swimming" signs posted around with warnings about some sort of bacteria.

It's a perfect, blue-sky, hot summer day. Hazel joins me. Jessica is running an errand. Summer wanders past, barefoot and walking tenderly. Smiling, she waves at us. We wave back. She takes off her yoga pants, stashes them under a bush and, blatantly disregarding the warning signs, wades into the murky green water. I suspect it's as green from pond scum as it is from duck feces.

"It's hot out today…but not hot enough to get me in that water," I say to Hazel.

"Hmm," she says, neither agreeing nor disagreeing.

Summer wades out farther as I try not to worry about the bacteria-ridden water giving her an infection where a girl least wants one. She dives, then surfaces, kicking and splashing. Indignant ducks quack and flutter away.

"So you live in Boston? Did you grow up around there?" Hazel asks.

"No, actually, I moved from Philadelphia after college—" I start to reply.

"May I join you?" Jaznae interrupts, appearing out of nowhere and already sitting down.

Again, that mysterious accent. Though the "inner essence" artist conversation from the first day lingers fresh in my mind, I say, "Sure. We were just talking about where we're from and where we live."

"I grew up in New York," Hazel says. "Then I moved to Cambridge for my master's and ended up staying."

"Oh cool. What about you?" I ask Jaznae in an effort to include her in the conversation.

"What? Because I'm black? I cannot be from here because I'm *black*? Well I *am* from Boston—ever since slavery ended. But because I'm *black*, you think I simply cannot be from here?!" Her tone is outraged, furious, attacking.

I'm totally caught off-guard. I assumed, reasonably I think, that she was not originally from Boston given her island-y accent. But in the face of this verbal onslaught, I stare helplessly at Hazel, who is poking at her salad with chopsticks. She doesn't appear to feel the need to defend herself or me. Clearly, she's gone to her happy place. I fervently wish I was there with her.

"No, I didn't mean...I was just asking...we were just talking about where we're from," I attempt stupidly, brain frozen in some sort of mire of white guilt and defensiveness.

Jaznae trills a phony laugh, as though I'm ignorant and that is somehow funny. "Just because I'm black doesn't mean I'm not from Boston."

"Well, *obviously*," I agree. "There are plenty of black Bostonians." To tell the truth, however, it didn't always feel that way. Coming from Philly, the sheer whiteness of downtown Boston, had, in fact, surprised me at first.

"We both moved here after college, so we thought maybe you did too," Hazel adds, in what I assume is a belated but welcome attempt to rescue this conversation. She turns as Janet walks up to us, then moves over to make room for her. I pray Janet's arrival will change the conversation altogether.

"Hey guys! Beautiful day out," Janet says, sitting down.

"College is a tool of the white man to keep the black man down," Jaznae says firmly, ignoring Janet's arrival and greeting. "I'm reading a book about Mother Africa and how all the skills we need come from the heritage of our people. Our heritage before slavery. Before the white man took it. College can't erase that. That is why I didn't go to college."

Janet looks from Jaznae to Hazel to me, clearly wondering what she just stumbled into. "Actually, that's simply not true," Janet says firmly. "Education is a tool that empowers everyone, regardless of race. I have my undergraduate and master's degree in education and I got them at a time when it wasn't easy for women or blacks to do either. But I did, and I went further in life because I did. And now I'm on the board of a local college. They really value diversity and want to make education available for everyone."

"I have all the education I need," Jaznae volleys back hotly. "I stay true to Mother Africa. I do not allow myself to be deluded by the man."

Janet looks away and starts to wrap up her lunch. "The purpose of education is not to delude, but to empower. I hope you'll understand that someday."

"I hope you'll return to truth!" Jaznae says churlishly.

"Okay. Well—time for me to head back!" I announce with forced lightness, shoving my half-eaten lunch back into my bag.

"Me too," Hazel adds, actually done. The three of us walk away, leaving Jaznae to sit by herself.

"That was intense," I say under my breath, still shaken.

Janet shrugs. "You can't let people like that get to you. She's clearly…wherever she is, and you can't let it get to you. Just…breathe it out."

"Hey guys! Wait up!" Summer calls, running to catch up with us, squeezing her hair out. Her white T-shirt is now a dingy greenish gray.

It's the last day of the immersion. "We're going to share our deepest scar with the group. We'll then write it on a scrap of paper and burn it to release it into the universe," Thea informs us.

Immediately a few of the yogis start crying. Harper, the grad student from Tennessee, bows her head on her folded arms and succumbs to outright sobs. The rest restrain themselves to delicate sniffles. I mentally retreat from the quickly escalating intensity.

Thea plows on regardless. It seems she forgot the ceramic dish that she cast specifically for this process, so today we'll use a plate she found in the studio's kitchen. "If you can heal and release the past, you'll have room and awareness in your life for new possibilities."

Um...isn't this what I'd done over countless martinis with girlfriends? I hated to think I'd wasted all that vodka.

Her voice warm and knowing, she continues. "If you can heal yourself, you can heal others." She pauses to let us absorb that. "*If* anyone wants to, they can opt out." Her voice, no longer warm, conveys that's not a good idea. And after that sizable lead-in about how to participate with the plate and the burning and the enhanced healing—and absolutely no information on how *not* to participate (leave the room? say "Pass!"? take child's pose?)—it seems inadvisable.

The silence in the room grows heavy. The pressure to confess instead of opting out grows in tandem. It feels like this will be a bonding experience. This is the first week of spending a year with these people, so if I opt out, and everyone else opts in, will I be on the "outs" for the rest of the year? The risk of social suicide seems too great. There's the additional detail of wanting to get all I can get out of this experience.

Thea turns toward me and my heart speeds up. "Let's start with this side of the room."

I have the extreme misfortunate of being seated in the first position. Everyone looks at me. I take a deep breath. "I stayed in a relationship with my ex-boyfriend for three years, even though he didn't treat me well. At the end, he was cheating on me with his secretary and everyone knew it but me."

It's been years, but I still wish with every bone in my body that I'd never put up with him in the first place. I should've told him to get the hell out of my life long before the cheating. I should've told him to go take a flying leap off the nearest bridge. No—I should've offered to assist him off the bridge with the hood of my car!

Thea nods but says nothing. I look at Summer on my left. It's her turn.

"My greatest scar is that sometimes I'm just *too* nice," she says, her voice utterly sincere.

I stop breathing. In the words of the venerated online community, *WTF?!* Now I feel stupid and vulnerable. Sort of like when my yoga friends Isabella and Julie had once suggested we have a "girls night in" of waxing.

As in, *wax hair removal*.

Tired of paying strangers untold amounts to yank out superfluous hairs at salons, Isabella had suggested, and Julie and I had agreed, it was more cost effective to simply buy the wax and do the deed ourselves.

The night arrived and the three of us sat around the microwaved container, looking at it dubiously. Rounds of, "You go first." "No, *you* go *first.*" "No, *you*," ensued until I agreed to *go first*. I doffed my jeans and took to the living room floor.

Very solemnly, they knelt on either side of me, hunched over my lower half and, in an homage to Mr. Miyagi in the original *Karate Kid*, "waxed on, waxed off," while I laid there, trying to feel fine about it.

When they were done, I leapt back into my jeans and grabbed the wax-laden popsicle stick. "Okay, who's next?"

Julie deferred, shaking her head. "I pluck my eyebrows, and I only wax my pubes in the summer."

"Lip? Brow? Underarms? Legs?" I offered.

"Nah. I'm all set. I'm really lucky—I'm not very hairy."

"Well, it's not like I'm '*hairy*'!" I protested, annoyance escalating at the sneaking suspicion that I'd been dogged out.

I turned to Isabella. "What are you going to do?"

"Oh, I'm all set. I waxed my own bikini line, legs, and brows earlier."

I was teetering on outrage. "*What?* I thought this was our girl's-night-in thing."

"Well, I do have like three hairs on my right big toe that I could do without," Julie offered, probably to appease me.

A freaking *toe? Really?* "You know what? Let's just forget it," I snapped.

Isabella obligingly waxed Julie's big toe while I tried not to pout.

Now, here I was, years later, and basically in the same situation. Summer had offered the equivalent of her big toe, and I was mad I'd bared it all.

Resolutely, I pull my attention back to the exercise. One by one, the rest of the trainees confess their deepest scars. Unlike Summer, everyone else confesses what I'd expected: the sort of wounds that can haunt people for the rest of their lives. As the confessions snake around the rest of the circle, secrets—the kinds of things that maybe even your really close friends don't know about you—pour out. And it is kind of bonding, because unlike the waxing incident, the rest of the yogis don't hang me out to dry.

Thea leads us in a final chant and dismisses us. I'm disoriented as I drive home. Like when you go to the movies in the middle of the day, completely lose track of the time, and emerge hours later, shocked to discover it's still light out. I've been so immersed in the rhythms of teacher training, that it will be a jolt to reenter the stratosphere of my real life.

In case I'm worried about going yoga-less, there is still all the homework to do. That night, as I slowly work through it, the question that really stumps me is defining and outlining my individual project. I think of Jaznae and Brinley. And even sweet, oblivious Summer with her drumming and her non-fear of germs and duck feces. If they're yogis, then I know for sure I'm not. I've never felt more corporate and strait-laced in my entire life. I—who usually feels like the alterna-girl in the corporate world—am now the conservative, uptight one. Not because I've changed, but because of the people I'm surrounded by.

Then it dawns on me: for my project, I'll attempt to integrate this duality—my inner straitlaced corporate stiff and my inner funky yogic tree hugger. I'll attempt to assimilate them and become an *urban yogini*. I won't renounce urban life to go dwell in a yurt and meditate all day. Neither will I let corporate life turn me into a nautical-themed, tie-wearing robot. I will become an utterly Zen being, sitting in lotus, untouched and unaffected by trifles like traffic and crowds.

I lean back, satisfied and proud. *Urban yogini*—I like how that sounds.

Chapter Nine

Meanwhile, Back at the Office...

How to Tell Someone They Stink

Monday morning, I arrive at work to find framed 8x10 shots of Vicky in a tiny sequin costume sprinkled throughout the office—on the credenza, the filing cabinet, by the copier. Everywhere I look, there she is, as featured in her community theater's latest production, in her tiniest costume yet.

The apocalypse is imminent. The only thing worse than *visualizing* your boss covered only by a few sequins held together by the equivalent of dental floss is actually *seeing* it. Now I've seen it. And what has been seen cannot be unseen. Sharklike teeth gleaming out at me. Painfully skinny body—bones barely covered with scarce dangly muscle. Jazz hands spread like raptor claws. Eyes wide with rabid glee.

When Vicky described her theatrical exploits, my imagination, with a strong instinct for self-preservation, always spared me this level of detail. For obvious reasons. The photographic reality, however, leaves little to the imagination. And what it does leave, I cannot allow myself to imagine.

I resolutely close my office door; time to shut myself back into my corporate life. I slip my suit jacket over the back of the chair—strange to be back in suits and heels after being barefoot and in comfy yoga clothes every day—and get down to work. In addition to an unfathomable backlog of to-dos, there's a slew of wedding-related voicemails: apparently, we need to find another rehearsal dinner venue because the restaurant we originally booked is closing unexpectedly, the photographer needs to scout the locations to determine lighting, and my future mother-in-law has left three messages with questions about what to stock the bathroom baskets with—a task I assigned her to help her continue to feel included. Additionally, there's a snafu with the hotels—guests are being told there are no rooms left even though I blocked more than enough. I've also just learned the church booked a wedding directly before ours and I'm worried about a wedding collision. Most important, I still haven't found shoes and have no time to go shopping.

Workwise, I'm holding the company's first press briefing in just a few weeks. This sort of big-splash event is the reason I was hired. My reputation and future success rides on the briefing's success. I need reporters from the crown-jewel media outlets to show up, nothing disastrous or newsworthy to scoop us, and, most of all, for it not to rain. Reporters will famously not show up if they have to battle the weather, even if you offer a fully catered breakfast at great expense to your budget, which I am. Within my control, there are hundreds of deadlines and decisions lurking and an unfathomable number of phone calls and emails to be returned.

With every task, I steadily reimmerse myself in the corporate world. The yoga world of the past week fades as though it was nothing more than a chimera, a dream that I'd willed to life for a bit. It's disorienting to be back in the office, but I firmly reground myself with the mundane. This is my life. This is the real world.

A few very productive hours later, I tap on my colleague Angela's door. She helps manage conferences, but has never been promoted to a title position. Given her inherently soft-spoken nature, she never will be. "Ready to go see Captain Theatrical?"

Angela rolls her eyes. "Ugh. I don't know if I'm up to it." As we reluctantly walk over to Vicky's huge window office, she trots alongside me, not letting the fact that she's six inches shorter and wearing stilettos slow her one bit.

We pause outside the glass walls of Vicky's office, waiting to catch her eye and get the nod to come in, but she's feverishly absorbed in her computer, intermittently pounding at the keyboard.

"She's posting the new pictures to her dating website," Betsy shouts over from her cube a few feet away.

I roll my eyes, and Angela and I barge in. "Vicky? Quick question: we've got the final proposals. Can you sign off?"

She doesn't look up. There is only a crusty remnant of her Soviet red lipstick left around her lips. "Can you come back later? I've really got to finish this. Angela said that men like women who have interesting hobbies. She said I should upload my theater pictures."

I shoot Angela a look and shake my head disbelievingly.

Angela's face is carefully arranged. I haven't seen anyone try this hard to look innocent since the four-year old I used to babysit, his face smeared with chocolate, had *sworn* that a bear had come in and taken one bite out of each of the cookies I'd baked and left cooling on the counter.

Vicky is still fully absorbed in her task. "So I found this great service," she says absentmindedly. "A wildlife refuge has a trained parrot that you can rent for your wedding to fly the rings up the aisle. Isn't that fantastic? People would be talking about that for years."

I wrestle myself away from a disbelieving snort of laughter. *Single, white, crazy lady seeks marriage-minded man. Must enjoy amateur theater pics and be open to parrot ring bearer. Sanity optional. Willingness to share meds a plus.* "Wow!" I say instead. The irony that she's looking for wedding services as I'm the one who's about to get married isn't lost on me. I shiver and decide to abandon the plan of having her actually review the documents. Clearly, she's not up to it. "So…can I just grab your signature and we'll be out of your way?"

"Just leave them. I'll get to them later."

Angela shrugs: *What can we do?*

I toss them on her desk and we leave.

As we walk past Betsy's desk I spin my finger in the air around my ear. "Cuck-oo! Cuckoo!"

"Tell me about it. And look at blondie egging her on." We both turn to Angela.

"Hey, if she's happier, maybe we'll be happier," Angela says.

"Maybe she'll even move away!" I add.

Betsy nods toward Vicky's office. "Her desperation is reaching an all-time low. She's all-out advertising with those shots all around the office, but so far, no nibbles—I've been checking her email. She's even flirting with the new guy from IT. Have you *seen* him? The guy needs a bra. No joke. He's got moobs."

The Meat saunters up. "Ladies," he drawls, giving us each the once-over and lingering unabashedly breast-high. "Looking good, *looking good.*" Reluctantly, he wrests his gaze upward. "Hey, Betsy, cover my phone while I'm out, will ya? I gotta hit up a little lunchtime shopping—upgrade the *pantalones.* Probably gonna set me back a few hundo, but I can only wear the pleat-front, if you know what I mean— plenty of room in the crotchal area." This is punctuated with a two-finger double point to his groin. "There's a reason they called me 'The Meat' in college."

There's a different reason we call you "The Meat" now, I think.

He winks. "I'm gonna crush the chicks this weekend."

We watch as he struts off down the hall. Betsy shakes her head sadly. "This place is a social tundra."

The weeks between the immersion and the next workshop churn in the usual grinding fashion—filled with work, maneuvering around Vicky's increasing instability, travel for work, yoga homework, the never-ending tasks inherent to wedding planning, and, in spare moments, trying to squeeze in a few dinners with Nunnally and some semblance of a life. And has anyone ever successfully "squeezed" in a life? In that amorphous "life" arena, my best friend came out of the closet, an unmarried friend found herself pregnant, and a married friend found herself fertility-challenged. Apparently, some people weren't just thinking about yoga or their jobs.

I get my homework back from Thea and skim to the end to read her response to my urban yogini idea. She writes about my anxiety as an outgrowth of long-standing neurological and neuro-emotional patterns (whatever those are) and suggests that I focus my yearlong project on a combination of *svadvaya,* self-study; *asana,* poses; and *pranayama,* breathwork to rebalance my nervous system. I scowl. *But what about becoming an urban yogini?*

In an attempt to keep me away from the office and to stem my "mutinous ways," Vicky sends me to management training. It's full of useful information such as the HR-approved method for telling employees that the foul stench of their unwashed bodies is distracting you and your co-workers. Apparently, it would be *wrong* to scream, "You stink, you filthy pig!" in front of other people in the break room. Thanks to the training, I now know that the *right* way to handle this situation is to tell him/her in private, "Listen, Joe/Jane. You're a valued employee here at the widget factory. But sometimes, the scent of your body is too strong." Three days of super useful information like this more than justifies the mountain of work that accumulates while I'm gone.

Back from the training, Betsy pops her head into my office. "Captain Theatrical wants me to tell you that she finds it inappropriate that you're showing off your boobs like that."

I glance down at my modest boatneck, culled on sale from my corporate staple, Banana Republic. If I was any more covered I could pass for a nun, but I'm nervous that she'll report me to HR for sexual harassment or some other imaginary infringement if I don't change. "What can I do?"

Betsy shakes her head resignedly. "You know how it is. Last week it was *my* dress—*I* was showing *mine* off. Week before that, it was the *receptionist* showing *hers* off. She's just jealous of anyone who actually *has* boobs. I told her to gain ten pounds."

What would I do without Betsy? "Seriously though, how do you do it? How have you lasted?" She's been here ten years. I could learn something.

Betsy chortles. "At least she doesn't throw staplers at my head like my last boss. But we've moved past that. I still have drinks with her."

I imagine Vicky throwing a stapler at my head. What would I do? Cry? Grab a keyboard and beat her down? Lunge at her with an animalistic snarl and settle this once and for all? Staple her lips to the wall? All seem possible. Drinks together, however, were definitely not an option. I shudder remembering the binge that led to the Great Upchuck Incident.

As though her ears are burning, Vicky suddenly pops up. She shoots a withering glare at Betsy. "I'm still waiting on those copies for my theatre workshop application," she says icily, "unless you're too busy chatting?"

"Ahh, missions like this take me back to my days at the FBI," Betsy says, rolling her eyes as she sashays away.

Vicky seems blissfully unaware of her sarcasm and zeroes in on me instead. "I didn't like how you were breathing at the meeting last week."

"Which meeting?" I ask before realizing that I shouldn't dignify an accusation about my *breathing* with a response.

"Oh please! You know which one. Friday's *obviously*. You were breathing rebelliously. You were trying to signal to everyone else that you should have my job. You…you're always plotting against me. You all are."

I freeze, terrified of what's coming.

But her mood turns on a dime and suddenly she's happy, genuinely unconcerned. "But it's okay! Everyone wants my job! Everyone wants to be me!" She laughs breezily.

If only my breathing could convey what I really think.

Chapter Ten

Preparing for the Zombie Apocalypse

Am I Wearing a Crazy Magnet?

I swing by Betsy's desk to pick her up for lunch. Spotting a potential audience, Vicky rushes over with a huge smile. "Girls!" she coos. "You will not believe what happened. Sara will really love this." She's laughing so hard she can barely get the story out.

"I was leaving the office and the cleaning people caught me taking a gallon of milk home from the break room! Can you *imagine*?! The cleaning people catching *me*! But what can I tell you? It makes so much more sense than me buying it. I just freeze it and thaw it a little bit at a time."

Betsy's mouth turns down at the mention of frozen milk.

Charles emerges from his office. "What's this?" he asks in his disapproving way.

Vicky, practically howling with laughter, drapes herself against him. "Charles!" she mock-scolds. "Were you listening to my funny little story?" She peers flirtatiously over her glasses at him.

"Vicky, really," he says, gently disentangling himself. "*Freezing milk? From the break room?* Are you trying to tell me something? Do we not pay you enough?"

I grit my teeth. She must rake in at least $500,000. Which is $499,999 more than her work's worth.

"You are just too much!" she squeals, delighted.

My efforts to finish the workweek on time fail, and I race the clock to get home. I quickly change into yoga gear as an external indication of the transition between corporate and yoga containers—or some such yoga-speak—and arrive at the training stressed from rushing and the long, traffic-filled commute. The irony of *rushing* to do yoga is not lost on me. I claim a seat against the wall next to Jessica. One valuable lesson from the immersion was that sitting next to normal people *and* against the wall is key to survival…of both the mental and physical bodies, as the yogis would say. I rip open a snack bar to tide myself over for the next few hours.

Thea brings the class to attention and leads off the chant.

As per usual, I can't settle in. I can't even seem to keep my eyes closed. I peek at Jessica. She's peeking too.

I chant quietly, trying to look yogic and mellow, like I blend in and belong here. But honestly, I just want to get back to my snack. I'm cranky, hungry, and tired, sort of like a two-year old, but taller.

On the positive side, at least I get to wear yoga clothes and be barefoot. It feels so decadent after being stuck in suits and heels.

Thea ends with a long "OM," then slowly looks around, considering. "It's important to recognize and accept, to observe with compassion, the mental chatter, especially in anxious people—without getting upset or angry at their inability to relax and be still in both the mental and physical bodies."

Is it my imagination or do her eyes rest an extra beat or two on me? I freeze guiltily, snack bar in hand. *How does she know about my mental chatter? Why can't I be one of these Zen yoga people?* I want to be like the lioness I saw on the Discovery Channel, basking languorously in the sun, the stress-free Queen of the Serengeti. But instead I feel like the anxious little vervet monkey hiding in the baobab tree, thoughts hopping around maniacally.

A lioness would pontificate wise idioms like, "Ahhhhh yes…recognize and accept…observe with compassion…." But instead I'm the human equivalent of a frenetic little primate and my mental track is more like, *How much longer until we can go home? It's Friday night. I'm tired. I'm hungry. Ooh—maybe I'll have pizza later* *and then some caramel swirl ice cream. I hope Picco isn't sold out. Caramel swirl goes fast. But wait, could the sugar keep me awake? Oh screw it. I'll counteract any energizing effects with a nice glass of red wine. Or two. Sugar and alcohol—two sins to hide from the yogis. Crap, what if they find out....*And on and on, a tiny little monkey's grand scheme for a schizoid, simian cosmos.

Thea continues. "In addition to learning poses, we're also going to explore breathwork, *pranayama,* this weekend, as a way of addressing mental body issues like anxiety or depression."

Even I—the non-yogi yoga student—know it's not an overstatement to say that breathing is kind of important. Forget using it as a tool to deepen your practice, you'll be lucky to get through the first two postures before you collapse in a heap on your mat if you forget to breathe properly. On a more advanced and esoteric level, *pranayama* is also employed to try and still the mind, prepare for meditation, and enhance internal awareness beyond the physical realm of *asana.*

At some point, after a lot of talk about breathing, Thea gives us a five-minute break. As is standard, in blatant disregard of the importance of her boundaries, much of the class stampedes towards her to bask in her Thea-ness or ask how what she just said applies to their tight hamstrings/energetic blockage/mother's emotional inaccessibility. Trying not to get elbowed or trampled, I step outside to get some fresh air. It actually scares me that I've gotten so used to the smell of sweaty feet and musty blankets that I only smell them when I first arrive, yet I know that I must be inhaling the stale odor the whole time. I breathe as deeply as I can to try to cleanse my lungs and aerate my brain.

When I return, the usual cluster of students are still standing around Thea like fans outside a stage door. *Surely, Thea must need a break too,* I think, recalling her endless discussion about the importance of boundaries. Maybe she wouldn't have such a dogged attachment to boundaries if her students respected them in the first place. Instead, Jessica and I seem to be the only ones to respect her invisible barbed-wire fences. The clamoring reminds me of an amped up herd of cattle. And as we all know, amped up herds will mow down anything.

Thea resumes her lecture, which is apparently the only thing that can send everyone scampering back to their seats, and we begin.

"The body holds physically what the mind holds mentally..." Thea intones.

Brinley's hand snakes up. "Will we be spending some time on the special needs of mothers? And also what parts of the body are more likely to hold certain 'stuff'—especially the spleen?"

Ah yes, now it's real. I'm back at yoga training.

"Feeling mentally supported has effects in the physical body. Just as feeling physically supported can help support the mental body. That's true for those of us who are mothers as well as those of us who are giving birth to ideas or nascent parts of ourselves. It's all connected in the world of mind-body medicine," Thea says.

She uses the answer to segue into her next lesson about how the effects of relaxation are deeply healing on every level of our being and how we're in for a treat this weekend. It's clear that all this mind-body stuff is her passion. Her eyes gleam and, for the first time since I've met her, she actually giggles. For a second, the stern boundary-driven taskmaster is gone and someone young, girlish, and playful has taken her place. But only for the briefest of moments. And then the lighthearted imposter is gone and the usual no-nonsense Thea is back.

Thea drifts in late again the next morning, the yoga sun in this universe. The energy of the room shifts around her, everyone focused entirely on her. "Restorative yoga can yield amazing releases and transformations," she begins. "I had a student who fractured a bone in her hand and her doctor said she needed to have surgery. But I suggested she put it off and do restorative yoga several times a week instead. And four weeks later, x-rays confirmed she wouldn't need surgery—her hand had completely healed on its own."

There is a predictable level of awe at this.

"But not everyone is going to be able to experience truly transformational, life-changing releases, so it's best not to talk about it so you don't set any expectations."

As though she herself had not just done this, Thea looks around the circle slowly, warningly, and I try to hide the fact that all I can think about is that I really want to have a life-changing release.

Thea pauses meaningfully. "The most significant transformations are internal shifts. How many times have you said, or heard other people say, 'I'm anxious,' or 'I'm depressed,' or 'This is me—that's just the way I am?' Well, restorative yoga can change all that by rewiring your brain and creating new neurological patterns."

I feel smarter even writing "new neurological patterns" in my notebook and I'm not even sure exactly what it means. But the idea of being able to change ourselves, of being able to literally reconfigure ourselves to be less anxious, less depressed, more relaxed, and happier—and all through a passive practice of yoga—is not just enticing, it's freaking awesome!

Thea hands out copies of a workbook. "I guess I'm still paying off that karmic debt to the copy place." She laughs. "Somehow my order got messed up again." She shakes her head, looking amused, as the class giggles adoringly. "So just flip through and switch the front and back pages, and then I'll hand out pages two, ten, and seven, because they came in this separate box for some reason."

Yogi disorganization follows. "Which pages are separate?" Summer asks.

"Switch which pages?" Gloria asks, massaging one of her feet with great vigor.

"Order is irrelevant. We need to meditate on *meaning*," Brinley says, palms clasped over her abdomen.

I shake my head and make the adjustments. All I know is that in my many, many dealings with various copy places, my order has never gotten messed up. Maybe I don't have a karmic debt. Or maybe I submit it in such an organized and exacting manner so as to be near impossible to mess up. I try to restrain myself from my obsessive-compulsive impulse to organize each one myself. I can practically feel beads of sweat break out on my forehead with the effort of not saying, "Just let me do it, for crap's sake!"

The workbooks include precise written instructions for every pose, along with stick-figure illustrations by an artist who, Thea informs us, traded this work for private sessions. "Community...community is a powerful, beautiful thing," she intones.

The entire room nods thoughtfully. "Community is so powerful," Kim echoes, looking especially blond and perky.

"I'm so thankful to be part of this community!" Gloria says, still massaging a foot.

"Community is the reason I took this training," Brinley adds definitively.

Thea smiles and nods at each of these affirmations. "So to get hands-on experience, we'll rotate partners to integrate the practice of teaching and assisting. As we do, let's be mindful of the practice of giving and receiving." Apparently, nearly everything in yoga is a practice.

We chant and partner up. And suddenly, as we get underway, this restorative yoga stuff seems quite challenging. Restorative yoga seems to consist of lying down on a mat and being entirely supported by blankets, bolsters, blocks, and straps. The variety and amount of propping customized to each person that every single pose requires is no small feat. Playing the teacher, I come face-to-face with my fear of touching random bodies because I rarely manage to get paired with my friends. Furthermore, I learn the hard way that body parts are surprisingly heavy when they're floppy deadweight.

Even if the student isn't large, a leg is surprisingly heavy. Trying to move two of them in a seamless, graceful way to ease the person into a pose while creating a sense of being cared for isn't easy. Sort of like steering a rubber wheelbarrow... through mud...on a rainy day...up a hill. As I flop one of Janet's arms into her own face, eliciting a startled, "What are you *doing*?!" and then proceed to accidentally drop one of her legs in the process of doing a required assist, I suddenly develop a tremendous appreciation for how challenging this work is.

To make matters worse, Thea seems to have a finely tuned talent for constantly popping up when you'd rather she didn't, while being nowhere to be found when you have a question. Knowing that she's probably witnessing every single fumble only serves to heighten my anxiety.

"The blanket goes lengthwise," Thea corrects me, appearing out of nowhere. I go to make the adjustment, but she takes an extra one and does it herself. Not being allowed to correct the mistake feels worse.

Thea glides toward Jaznae, who is working nearby. "What else do you think this practitioner could use?" Thea asks, eyeing Jaznae's extensive handiwork.

"Nothing!" Jaznae says proudly. "She is perfect."

I glance over. Jaznae's student is no longer visible—I pray it's not Jessica—as Jaznae apparently commandeered eight additional bolsters and propped them like an A-frame house around her student.

"Let's take another look," Thea says firmly as she deconstructs the bolster fort.

I look down at my partner. Janet is resting on her back in supported *savasana*, with a bolster under her knees, two blankets folded lengthwise under her spine, an extra blanket under each arm from shoulder to fingertips, and the one Thea painstakingly folded for her over her abdomen. She looks so vulnerable, lying supine, eyes covered with an eye pillow. She's in a sea of similarly resting bodies with student teachers micro-adjusting their props. I step backward and hear the sickening crunch at the same time that I register I'm stepping on flesh-covered bone. I move quickly, but not quickly enough.

"Owww!" Gloria howls rightfully, jerking up to a seated position and sticking her fingers in her mouth. "Ow, ow, ouchies!" These last iterations come out garbled around the injured digits.

"I'm so sorry!" I gasp, appalled at my own clumsiness. "Are you okay?"

Gloria and her teacher-partner stare indignantly at me.

Thea materializes out of nowhere. "One of our greatest lessons, as teachers and assistants, is that we need to be very mindful of where our bodies are in space as we work with a class."

"I'm so, so sorry," I repeat, mortified.

Janet and I switch roles and I quickly realize that, as a student, the work is strangely difficult as well. Unexpectedly, it's hard to tell if you're comfortable or not, if you just need a moment to settle into the pose or if it's truly not working for your body. It's also hard to identify the source of your discomfort or how it might be eased. Yes, your chest may feel like it's being squashed into the bolster, and you may want to reflexively cram a pillow under it, but what actually alleviates your discomfort may be more height under the shoulders and head, or less height under the hips, or a lower bolster, or an extra bolster.

Once you do find the ever-elusive complete physical comfort you then face the Herculean task of trying to turn off your busy-bee brain. To stop thinking about how you need to remember to get milk on the way home, or if you returned that phone call, and what that co-worker really meant when she said, "Whatever... I guess it's fine."

On some deep, guilt-harboring level, it's also tough to allow yourself to wholly receive care from another person—especially if that person is someone who you barely know, who isn't a friend, family member, or an anonymous massage therapist or aesthetician who you've paid to attend to your muscles or clogged pores, but simply a fellow teacher-trainee. I don't want to seem too demanding or high-maintenance. I worry I'm taking too long. Perhaps most ridiculous, I'm afraid my partner's next partner will be better at this relaxing business. One thing is for sure: this restorative yoga stuff—the yoga of nonaction—is far more complex than it seems at first glance.

Finally, Thea gives us a break. Summer plunks herself down in the middle of the room, opens a crumpled brown paper bag and pulls out a head of celery. She rips off a stalk and starts eating it, unwashed and unaccompanied. Brinley asks another student to help her get into the last pose we practiced. Of course, it's the most complicated, requiring seven assists and every prop known to yogadom. Gloria walks over and watches intensely, as though this is the most fascinating and important thing she's ever seen. Jaznae makes a show of announcing that she must rest in a pose for female energy because her cycle is really working her over. "Maybe it's the equinox," she says, pausing for effect.

The rest of the weekend consists of more of the same: receiving and administering the poses.

I'm folding a blanket, about to prop Jessica, when Thea is suddenly at my elbow. I freeze.

"Good!" she says, nodding at my work. "Nice, Sara!" Then she's gone.

I'm so shocked at the praise that I forget what I'm doing. I try not to focus on the fact that it's only a tidbit of praise for being able to fold a freaking blanket.

"So…one thought about group projects," Thea calls as we're about to go on one of the too-few breaks. "While we're following our own organic paces, remember it's never too early to start. So might I suggest that we spend our break time finding our group partners. Arrange however you want, any number of group members, any number of groups."

Mass chaos ensues. Twenty-two yogis-in-training start milling about, talking to their nearest neighbors. This basically equals a yoga cacophony.

Janet wanders over to me. We decide it'll be easiest for us to meet and work together, since we both live in the South End. Several others stop by, but keep moving when they realize we're Boston-centric. Kim, the blond psychologist, joins us, and I wonder if we can curtail the group at three. But before I can voice this thought—and frankly because I'm afraid of seeming exclusive and un-yogic—I see Jaznae heading straight for us. I stiffen nervously.

"And what group is *this*?" she demands.

"The South End Boston group," Janet answers.

"Perfect! I will be in this one."

My heart sinks.

"So…where and when shall we meet, ladies? I live on the other side of the river, out past Cambridge, so let's be mindful to choose somewhere close to me."

"Well, we were thinking somewhere in the South End—" Janet starts to say.

Jaznae cuts her off. "I suggest we meet closer to where I live, as that will be best for me. My art studio will be perfect."

"That seems like a good option," Kim says.

Annoyed by Kim's acquiescence, I look longingly toward Jessica and Hazel's groups. But by now all the yoga shuffling is done, and people are standing in definitive knots. I can't think of a socially acceptable reason to jump ship and cross the infinite length of the room. So instead I stay silent and remain rooted to where I am, mired in the unique and terrible feeling of being trapped with a lunatic. Unfortunately, the feeling is all too familiar.

Chapter Eleven
Some Things Shouldn't Be Licked...

...Or Laid on Your Mat

Charles walks into my office, clutching my formal request to take time off for our honeymoon. "You can't miss the conference on the 15th!" he says. "Can you do a quick detour to New York and then back to your honeymoon?"

"And leave Nunnally alone in Italy?" I ask, appalled.

"I'm sure he'll understand," Charles says smoothly.

I take a deep breath and ignore my instinct to cave. "I'm sorry, but I really can't. We've both agreed to take time off...*for the first time in five years*." I try to sound stern.

Charles ignores this. "Think about it," he says as he leaves.

The Meat strolls in, high-fives Charles as they pass, and plops down in my guest chair. He throws his feet up on the desk and gestures to my monitor which has slid to screensaver mode. It's a picture of Nunnally and me. "*Niiiice*," he says with a chuckle. Embarrassed, I quickly jiggle the mouse to make it disappear. He grins. "So....What's going on? Got any treats?" My snack drawer is legendary on our floor.

"Would you mind getting your freaking feet off my desk?" I ask, still rattled.

"Oh, DiVello," he chortles, throwing his head back. "Di-Vel-lo. Whaddaya—afraid of germs or something?"

"Do you ever think about what you step in just on your way here?'

"Please. I drive," he says, implicitly reminding me that once you're a VP, you get a garage spot, a huge perk in any city, but especially in Boston where parking is a competitive sport. "Anyway, you worry too much. I never worry. In fact, I'd lick the bottom of my shoes." He wiggles his eyebrows at me.

I lean back in my chair and cross my arms. "Do it."

His face lights up. "You don't think I'll do it? I will…for five bucks."

I reach for my purse—*Please God, let me have a five*—and slap the money on the desk. Bluff called. "Betsy! Get in here!" I yell.

Betsy walks in just as The Meat takes off his left shoe, turns the sole toward the sky, and takes a good, long lick. He leaves a wet swath behind.

"Ew!" Betsy says, "That's disgusting!"

"Worth every penny," I say.

As part of our training, Thea also required us to take at least one class with her outside the scope of our weekend workshops. It was a semi-return to the casual class-taking that I'd enjoyed so much back when I was just a student and not a student-teacher-trainee.

Theoretically, it makes sense to require us to practice outside workshops since the workshops themselves don't provide any actual yoga. But in reality, working this job makes it somewhat harder to drag my weary ass to Thea's midweek class. And, perhaps more important, evening classes push dinner back.

Thus, I resentfully find myself in her Wednesday evening class, where I mulishly plop my mat in the back row. Previously, yoga had been my place of refuge and respite. Now, between the perpetual workshops, ensuing self-study, homework, and the required class, yoga was starting to feel strangely like work. And we hadn't even gotten to the 40 hours of assisting, or group or individual projects yet.

With a sigh, I pull the tube of my mat out of its holster and with a swift flick of my wrists unfurl it in front of me. Somehow just seeing its warm, welcoming length makes me feel a smidge better.

At some indiscernible point, the process of stepping onto the mat had become ceremonial. My mat served as a physical gateway to a mental, spiritual, and emotional oasis—a welcoming island in the midst of the wasteland of my professional career and the labyrinth of the dilemma I'd fondly termed "my one-third-life crisis."

I once heard a teacher describe yoga as an opportunity to breathe out whatever you needed to "into the ever-loving receptacle of your mat." I couldn't agree more. My mat was an endlessly spacious vessel that could absorb anything, and make pretty much everything better.

Although sometimes I worried that it might run out of capacity—that I was overdumping my emotional crap into it—and that like any septic tank it would eventually run out of room and overflow my own refuse back at me. This was an unpleasant possibility to contemplate. So sometimes during an especially stressful day at work, when I'd been driven to the outer limits of my tolerance or abilities, I would grab my mat, stashed safely under my desk along with a rather large variety of high heels, and force myself to leave the bonds of my desk and escape to a lunchtime class.

There, I would step carefully onto it—always respectfully, always with reverence—and assume child's pose. Resting back on my heels with my forehead down, I'd place my palms carefully *off* the mat, flat on the floor, and purposefully breathe out my latest trouble, co-worker, client, or deadline into the oak. I figured the floor, with its wonderful fibrous nature and earthy origins, had much greater capacity for absorption than my comparatively tiny rectangular refuge. Plus, I had to protect my poor, overburdened mat. I was worried it couldn't handle my life. Its celestial nature had thus far proved to be infinite, endlessly abundant. More so than wine, dark chocolate, or nachos, it was keeping me sane. I couldn't lose that.

As I'd exhale my day, I'd think horrible, completely un-yogic thoughts like, *I'm leaving you here, Vicky, you wine-guzzling loon. In fact, all you squashed turds at Invest-o-crap. You're not going to get me down. I won't let you.*

Pushing aside thoughts of squashed turds and wine-guzzling loons, I step onto the mat on this particular night and transition instantly from the mindset of resentment over how much of my precious free time the training and its requirements are consuming to one of gratitude for this peaceful escape from work stress.

And if my thoughts stray inadvertently to concerns about what to eat for dinner and if I'll actually be able to relax and be worry- and thought-free in class, those concerns are swiftly assuaged by Thea's deft guidance through the drop-in and *pranayama*. As always, her teaching is brilliant.

Like the Pied Piper, she leads the class into a place of stillness in both body and mind, weaving a web that catches us as we fall into the deepest parts of ourselves. *That's so insightful,* I think several times as I marvel at her uncannily accurate verbiage, urging us to let go, release, explore…but I know I won't be able to remember what she said later.

On her cue, I open my eyes slowly, reemerging from the tranquil depths of inner stillness. It feels like I'm dragging my consciousness up from the bottom of the Caribbean Sea—the warm, turquoise water is a welcoming womb for my tightly clenched, overanxious brain. I smile groggily, already peaceful, and we haven't even begun the physical practice yet. At this point, I don't want to. I want to breathe and sit here some more. But alas, that time is behind us.

As we begin active practice, I dig deep to find the energy to hold the poses. I'm on day nine of work without a break. We flow from sun salutations, *surya namaskaras*, into warrior, *virabhadrasana*, and eventually land in garland pose, *malasana*, a deep squat.

I settle in, trying to let my heels reach for the floor while not toppling backward and landing on my tush. My lower back unclutches after a long day.

Thea speaks of breathing, and I deepen my breath to join with the rest of the class in deep cadenced *ujjiy*. We are one rhythmic machine. We breathe in and out in unison to spark our endurance, support our bodies, and circulate *prana*—life-force energy.

Suddenly, a loud fart rips through the air. It wasn't a high-pitched squeak as though the owner had tried to prevent its escape. It wasn't abbreviated as though the perpetrator had managed to wrest control over it midflight from its take-off point of anal origin. No, it was tubalike. Triumphant. Full-bodied. It was one of the most unabashed expressions of flatulence I'd ever heard. Not that I was an authority. I'm a female. We don't *fart*.

I'm so startled, I nearly fall out of the pose. I look to my left, where it seemed to originate, and find a woman in her late 40s studying her mat as though her life depends on it. *Guilty,* I think, though she's so studious, so very *mindful,* that I actually consider for a moment that perhaps I imagined the entire incident.

To give her some privacy, I direct my gaze back to my own mat and reignite my deep breathing, which I had let totally lag due to my shock. I worry for a moment that perhaps I'm now inhaling her methane straight into my lungs, into my very being, a concerning idea regarding anyone's ass-gas, let alone a complete stranger's, but really what choice do I have? I keep *ujjiy* going.

We transition out of *malasana* and into the same sequence on the right side. Just as we enter *parsvakonasana,* extended side-angle pose, I hear my gassy neighbor emit another thunderous blast. Although this follows by mere minutes on the heels of her first discharge, it's still such a social anomaly that it startles me into twisting around to stare at her in surprise. This time, however, my curious gaze is met with one of equal hostility from her.

Yeah. I farted. Twice. And I'll do it again—this time directly into your freaking face if you don't play along, she seemed to be mentally telegraphing to me.

Since we'd twist toward her in the next pose, I play it safe and avert my eyes. But no sooner do I drop my gaze than I hear her tear ass a third time—this one louder and longer than any previous emission and followed by a delighted little sigh of contentment. There was no disguising this one. Everyone ahead of us turns around to stare. To my horror, the perpetrator immediately turns to glare indignantly at *me.* Then she looks down at her mat and shakes her head in apparent disgust.

I'm scandalized by her deception. Then I feel myself redden as all the shocked faces turn my way and eyebrows shoot up. *Nooooo!* I want to say. *It wasn't me! She's the tooter!* I want to clear the air so to speak, but instead I freeze, helpless and shamed.

Somehow I know that if there is an unapologetically flatulent person in a group setting of any kind in the future, then that person is always—*always*—going to seek me out.

Chapter Twelve
This Yogini Is a Bride

Eating in Italy

The wedding day dawns, miraculously sunny and warm. I'm barely awake after five hours of sleep, procured only through the grace of prescription meds, and just starting to contemplate procuring coffee and a bagel, when my cell phone buzzes. It's my almost-mother-in-law. "The hairdresser isn't here. The salon is locked. What should I do?"

A shiver of anxiety runs through my gut. I've scheduled back-to-back appointments with my favorite stylist for the bridesmaids, myself, and Nunnally's mom. She's scheduled to go first. I reach for the spreadsheet I created to track everything, wondering where the hell Rodrigo is. If he's late to start, we'll all go down like a row of dominoes. Then I glance at the clock and relax. "You're an hour early."

"Oh, I know," she says. "I don't like to be rushed."

I grit my teeth. "I'm sure he'll be there on time, but you can call me back if he's not."

In the time it takes to say goodbye, I get texts from my sisters who want to know where to park, my cousin who wants to know where to buy a curling iron, and Nunnally who forgot the rings and is sending the best man over to retrieve them. The doorbell blares like a high-pitched foghorn (who the hell thought that was a good idea?) and I buzz up the bouquet delivery.

This sets the tone for the frenzy of the day. After a flurry of hair and makeup appointments, the bridesmaids come back to our apartment to get dressed. Crowded with bags, bouquets, and styling products, it's never felt smaller. I don't mind at all. My aunt Joan carries the dress into the living-room-turned-temporary-bridal suite like an offering, her arms extended straight out in front of her and the length of beaded white silk across them. The bridesmaids part to make way, paying due homage to the hand-stitched artistry. She places the hem down and the swath pools like a silk origami rose. I step into the center. She pulls it up with a rustle and zips me in. The bridesmaids watch and, always self-conscious, I blush.

My uncle Martin picks me up in a limo and we drive to the meticulously landscaped Public Garden, a park on the border of Boston's Back Bay and Beacon Hill neighborhoods. Established in 1837, it was the first public botanical garden in America. Full of whimsically meandering paths, stately centuries-old trees, and perfectly manicured beds of flowers that the city changes out every few weeks, it's the perfect picturesque location for photos with bridesmaids. Apparently, I'm not the only one who thinks so: tourists stop and take pictures of us. *This is totally surreal*, I think.

The surrealism doesn't end there. The limo brings us to the church. I wait in the back as the bridesmaids process ahead of me. Then it's my turn and I think I actually stop breathing as I walk slowly down the aisle with my uncle Martin. Everyone watches us. My legs shake. Uncle Martin, at 6'9", is reassuringly steady and strong as we finally make it down the endless length to Nunnally.

Some brides have told me they don't remember the ceremony at all, but I'm hyperaware of every single sight and sensation, from the pungent smell of incense in the summer-warm air to the softly filtered light as it slants through the huge stained glass windows. *It's the yoga*, my brain whispers. Yoga is teaching me how to be present, how to tune in. This is one of the best rewards of my time on the mat, yet it's happening off the mat.

A few weeks ago, Father Bob had asked us to write letters about why we wanted to marry each other. I had assumed it was some sort of pre-wedding test to see if we were serious and mature enough to really get married. But unexpectedly, he quotes part of mine now, "Because Nunnally sees me for exactly who I am…and loves me anyway." Everyone laughs, and the sound echoes in the cavernous, marble space. Caught off guard—it wasn't a wedding test?—I feel exposed. If I had known they were going to be part of the ceremony, I would've been more poetic and less honest. Revealed now in front of the people I love most in the world, I laugh too, even as my heart kind of hurts and hot tears well up. I look down and focus on breathing.

The ceremony continues. Time is compressed and yet endless…kind of like *savasana* at the end of a class. Eventually, Father Bob pronounces us married. Nunnally kisses me, his full lips soft and familiar, and I hug Father Bob, feeling his short, scratchy beard. We process out into the bright sun; I'm dazed…and married.

Time accelerates as soon as we get to the reception. My sister Annie has selflessly offered to be in charge of our 95-year-old Nana and her 97-year-old sister, Auntie Evelyn. The ancient duo, fearless with the assistance of their walkers, give Annie a run for her money. They are tireless, eating, talking, and wheeling through the party, just as I hoped they would. Hanna, with a white orchid tucked into her riotous dark curls, shyly keeps her distance from the dance floor, instead talking with cousins who live far and wide.

Of course, not everyone is so quiet and calm. I'm reapplying lip gloss and chatting with my Aunt Joan when I suddenly hear the unmistakable thready strains of the Hava Nagila, which is somewhat unexpected since neither Nunnally nor I is Jewish. I look to the dance floor and see Nunnally on a chair being bounced jerkily in the air. "We're looking for the bride," the DJ announces on the mic. I shrink back against the nearest wall as a knot of groomsmen surge toward me. "No!" I shriek, terrified of heights and of falling. "Oh, go for it," my aunt says. "This is great!"

Still terrified, I'm boosted into the air as well. I white-knuckle clutch the seat of my chair and pray I don't fall off. And, that if I do, I won't be visibly bruised or bloody for the sake of the pictures.

"Was this your idea?" I ask my Russian-Jewish college roommates when I'm back on the ground, after what seems like an eternity in the airborne chair, heart still racing.

"I wish!" one says, pointing to the real culprit, who is cackling wildly in the corner. It's Ted, our most mischievous WASP friend from Vermont. "It's not a wedding until you have the Hava Nagila!" he says. Nearby, his wife Patti shakes her head and sips her wine.

Not to be outdone (I learned in my years of rooming with them that the Russians dearly love a challenge), a few minutes later, my roommates escort me out to the lobby, then thrust me into a closet and lock the door, thus introducing me to a fun cultural tradition they have that roughly translates to "hide the bride."

"*Nyet!*" I insist, utilizing my conversational Russian, which I picked up while living with them, and pounding my fist on the door. "*Eto* no fun!" Of course, it's even less fun when you're the one in the closet, the American groom doesn't know he must sing for his bride's freedom, and the rest of the guests have absolutely no clue what's going on but haven't seen the bride since she went to the bathroom half an hour ago.

Finally, the Russians, realizing Nunnally isn't going to come to this realization alone, inform him of his mission, and Nunnally gamely attempts a rescue serenade with the assistance of several groomsmen backup singers.

The rest of the evening passes in a blur of music, drinks, and dancing. "Everyone we love in one place at one time!" I marvel. Nunnally squeezes my hand.

As the last guests shuffle—and in some cases stagger—out after the last dance, we load up our car with leftover centerpieces and our engagement photo decorated with signed well wishes from guests. Nunnally closes the trunk and gives me hug.

"Married," I say. It still doesn't feel real.

The next day, we fly to Italy, a mutually agreed upon location based on our love of food and history, in that order. It's our first trip in over five years. We start in Santa Margherita, where we lie on trademark European beach chairs and listen as the ocean laps at the rocky shore, the sizeable pebbles making the sound of rain as they roll against each other with the tide. We swim out to a large inflatable raft and I'm surprised by how sharply cold the Northern Italian waters are in September. I climb out shivering, covered in goose bumps, and stay on the beach for the rest of the week.

Every night, we stroll around the town's quaint winding streets and eat home-made pasta and seafood that's so fresh we know it's only hours old. The pesto, traditionally made of basil, pine nuts, olive oil, garlic, and parmesan cheese, is so smooth and creamy that I'm sure they substitute cream for the nuts. I ask and they assure me no. Still, I wonder, how they got it to such a lush consistency. We eat it nearly every lunch and dinner. I could eat it every hour.

After we decompress in the sun for a week, we're ready to leave the slower pace of shoreline life. We take the train to Florence, with a brief pit stop in Piza, where Nunnally insists on having pictures taken of him in various poses "holding up" the Tower. I grimace and obligingly take them. "Stop pretending to strain," I tell him.

In Florence, we accidentally stumble across what I will conservatively estimate to be the most fantastic restaurant in the entire world. Located on the outskirts of the peppermint-striped *duomo*-centric bustle, *Il Profeta* is owned and operated by Claudio and his German wife Martina and has food of such a delicious and divine nature that we gravitate back there most nights. We try other establishments, of course, in an effort to be open-minded, but nothing compares to the delicate and yet robust flavors at *Il Profeta*.

"Very simple," Claudio says, modestly. "Not fancy. It's the ingredients. Very fresh. Come and learn."

I get teary as I eat a handmade pasta dish with a red sauce that reminds me of Nana's cooking, high praise indeed. I decide we should accept their kind offer to come and learn. Nunnally half-heartedly reminds me of our life at home.

Reluctantly, we leave *Il Profeta*, and not-so-reluctantly, we also leave the frenetic crowds, long lines of sweaty tourists, and hot stifling air of the city for the countryside in southern Tuscany.

There, for the first and last time, we rent a car and attempt the challenge of driving in Italy. We are assigned an impossibly tiny red two-door affair and putt-putt our way around. I would like to be able to say that we zoomed—just as I'd like to be able to claim I drive a standard and run a seven-minute mile—but none of these is remotely true.

Instead, our tiny car groans as Nunnally maneuvers it up the steep and treacherously winding roads that carve their way through olive groves and vineyards—both of us coaxing "Tiny Red" verbally as much as physically, and both of us equally concerned that I might have to get out and push.

As tiny as "Tiny Red" is—and the fact that only one of our suitcases fits in the trunk, despite mine easily meeting standard airline carry-on size limits, should give you an idea of just *how* tiny, she's proportionate to the Italian roads. Counting both lanes, the roads seem barely ten feet wide.

Local drivers, many in speedier, larger cars, literally zoom around the countryside with an admirably (or perhaps idiotically) blatant disregard for both speed limits and safety. As we inch our way along the narrow roads, hugging the middle of the road so as to be as far as possible from the cliffs with no guardrail, there is inevitably a line of cursing, impatient drivers behind us who lean on their horns and then speed past us in the oncoming lane. Although the driving is harrowing, it's hard to care, given that *we're driving through the Tuscan countryside.* Green rows of grape vines stretch across the rolling landscape. Days are long and slow and warm. The guidebooks are right: the light is incredible.

I look out the window and my mind wanders unwillingly to the fact that I'm missing the first meeting for my group project. Secretly, I'm relieved to miss it. Jaznae had already appointed herself as the boss and hijacked the project, insisting that we create a one-page form that can be used to create class sequences. My concern that sequencing is a topic we haven't yet covered—and won't for months—went unacknowledged. It seemed Janet and Kim didn't care enough to voice protest. Or maybe they lacked the radar I'd honed in my corporate tenure to discern bullshitters, imposters, and bad leaders. Whatever the underlying reasons, I found myself a hostage on the bad-idea express, bound for no glory. I was only too happy to be in Italy, far away from it all.

Tiny Red groans her way up the mountain back to our hotel. Between Nunnally, the reluctant driver, and me, his reluctant passenger-navigator, I'm not sure who was more relieved to return Tiny Red, albeit with some nostalgia, to the gas station where we rented her (which offers a cafe inside and vending machines for ice cream, chocolate, and condoms outside).

Before we know it, we're back in Boston, slightly dazed, but happy to be home. Even traveling for pleasure, on our honeymoon no less, to a place I'd yearned to go for years doesn't dim my homesickness for my own bed and little *appartamento.* Unfortunately, the *appartamento* reeks of now-moldy centerpieces and stale air. I open the windows, gather the flowers into giant trash bags, and try to ignore the tendrils of anxiety that snake into my belly when I think about going back to work. *Real life has to resume at some point,* I tell myself.

The next morning, I stride into the marble lobby among the usual rush-hour hordes. The staccato of heels on marble mixes with the baseline thunderous roll of conversation. I swipe my pass and the gate beeps its electronic permission. I exhale, worried as I always am, that I've been fired and that this is how I'll find out—being denied entrance at the security gates. This snafu would then hold up the endless lines of rushed, irate people trying to stream in behind me, ratcheting up to complete public humiliation.

In reality, this is a ridiculous worry based wholly on chronic anxiety and an unfounded fear of being homeless. Like every other day, I sweep through to the elevators that will whoosh me up to Investorcap. Like the other elevator occupants, I stare at the tiny screen with the day's headlines so that we don't have to contrive chitchat.

The doors ping open at Investorcap's floor and I make my way down the hall to my office. The dry, papery smell of endless reams of new paper and the greenish fluorescent light that seem to be an innate part of every office, pull me back faster than anything could. My windowless office seems especially dreary. My inbox has over 1,000 emails. Stacks of projects to be brought up to speed litter my desk. My voicemail box is at capacity. I suddenly remember why I haven't taken a vacation in over five years. Anxiety mixes with hopelessness and I try not to cry or hyperventilate. There's no chance of catching up—my upcoming travel schedule can only be described as insanity laced with lunacy, served with a side of madness.

"Look at that glow on your face after a few weeks in Italy…ah, newlyweds," Betsy says as she breezes by my office. "Come talk to me in a few years when you're stain-sticking his underwear, and he's swigging a beer and belching on the couch." Her chortle of a laugh drifts over her shoulder.

I laugh. In spite of the rest of this place, I'd missed her.

Chapter Thirteen:

A Case of the (Nine-Dollar) Crabs

Yoga Power & Other Mysteries

Back when the headhunter had first sent me the Investorcap job description, I'd liked that significant travel was required. *Excellent!* I'd thought, elated; *I love to travel!* It would be a chance to escape the desk shackles and explore the world on the company's dime, which included business-class flights and nicer hotels than I could afford. Most of all, it was a chance to escape the cubicle I'd been sitting in all day, every day, for years on end.

Studying abroad in college had served as the veritable first bite by the travel bug. Packing everything I owned into one very large backpack and heading overseas sophomore year had ignited a lifelong, never-ending desire to venture anywhere and everywhere. But perhaps most of all, I had always dreamed of traveling to India...a desire that had only intensified now that I was dipping a toe into the yoga world. Travel to the mothership was revered almost as much as foregoing formal housing in favor of living in a yurt. Or wearing swirly, organic hand-woven hemp. Or using the word "journey." A lot.

Regardless, the fact that Investorcap had offices in Southeast Asia had seemed like a sign at the time. I wanted to see new countries, learn about their histories, try their languages, and, of course, dive into their local cuisine. Have I mentioned that I like to eat? A lot? Sort of like I like to breathe?

Almost immediately after signing the acceptance letter, packing up my cube in the financial district skyscraper and moving a few short blocks away where I un-packed in a disappointingly similar skyscraper, I yearned for my first trip.

I'd imagined I would glide through the airport in a smartly tailored suit, high heels clicking efficiently, leather *attaché* swinging in rhythm with my every step. I'd slide into my luxe, oversized, first-class seat, sip white wine, and, looking very important, would review very important industry reports briefing me on the very important goals of the very important trip. Finally, feeling *très importante*, I'd settle in to enjoy the flight to some unknown and exotic location where, after completing the obligatory morning business meeting, I would spend the afternoon soaking in the local sights and then dining in a fabulous restaurant.

Which is why, you may understand, I was somewhat dismayed when my first trip was only to New York, and I'd spent the better part of it taking care of Vomiting Vicky.

Since then, most trips had been similarly un-fun. In keeping with my fantasy, my next one brings me to unknown and exotic suburban New Jersey. Thankfully, Vicky isn't coming. Instead, I'm accompanying the SVP of Conglomerate Synergization. Vomiting is optional.

We arrive at an office park and head into an outdated suite with threadbare carpets. The office has the empty, gloomy feel of a company going out of business. As the meeting begins, I prepare to take notes on brilliant, impending PR projects. But I soon realize, to my confusion and dismay, that this meeting has absolutely *nothing* to do with *anything* that I do. The purpose instead appears to be to prepare for the change from current senior management to the incoming team.

The outgoing group, who co-founded the company together 30 years ago, no longer speak to each other. The only thing they agree on is that nobody wants to retire or assist the new team in taking their places. This creates an interesting dynamic as we cram all four nonspeaking founders and all four incoming, resented, younger team members into one conference room to discuss the specifics of the hand off. The only thing all eight of them can agree on is that nobody wants the heavy-handed parent company coming in to tell them how to do anything. Cut to hostility toward the SVP and me.

I try to look interested, yet unobtrusive.

I wonder why I've been sent here.

I fantasize about a dramatic escape. Would that crawl-through-HVAC-vents thing you see in movies really work?

Five hours later, the meeting ends and one cantankerous 65-year-old founder, the outgoing CFO, drives several of us to dinner in his silver Jaguar. We arrive at the steakhouse and a valet approaches.

"How much is this gonna cost me, young man? Five dollars? Five dollars?" the CFO bellows. "That's ridiculous! Parking should be free!" He peels away and drives to a nearby mall parking lot. In his Jaguar. Over five dollars.

I don't complain that it's raining and we have no umbrellas, or that my fabulous new high heels excruciatingly erase skin from my heels as we hike the approximately 5,000 miles back to the restaurant.

We're the last to arrive at dinner, where we're reconvening with the rest of the outgoing team members. Several rounds of drinks lowers the hostility level down to a tolerable simmer. As we drink—high-end scotch for them and vodka tonics for me, as drinking anything more feminine would be career suicide but I hate scotch—I smile and nod as conversation progresses from baseball, to football, and finally to hunting. I have nothing to add.

Finally, conversation lulls. "So," I say, trying for casual, "have you guys given any thought to portable alpha?" It's a term I've been hearing a lot about lately and while I can recite the technical definition—something about "porting" alpha, extra returns, over the beta, market risk—I don't actually understand it. Understanding, however, is vastly overrated in the corporate world. All you really have to do is sprinkle a buzz word at the appropriate time and you've bought yourself some time and street cred.

The guy next to me raises his brows—*There's a female present! She speaks! She said portable alpha!*—and then the conversation ball is in play and I return to my smile-and-nod campaign.

A few more rounds and the guys are finally ready to order. The waiter announces there's one entrée special—steak Oscar. I perk up. Is there anything better than a high-quality, pasture-finished, perfectly proportioned filet mignon, lightly seasoned, and cooked to a precise medium rare? If there is, it's steak topped with crab.

"For the lady?" He turns to me, the only female at the table.

"I'll have the special," I say, mouth already watering.

My jaguar-driving chauffeur stares at me coldly, the lights overhead reflecting off his bald, shiny scalp. "That's nine dollars more than the filet!" he says indignantly, glancing around the table for support.

The positivity from the portable alpha moment vanishes. Everyone's suddenly extremely busy examining their menus.

My face turns red. Is nine dollars too much? I'm the only woman here—I don't want to draw any more attention to that fact. Oh, dear God. What should I do? Remind this pint-sized geezer that the parent company is picking up the tab? Retract my order? Or go down with the ship over a nine-dollar crab?

I glance at the SVP for guidance but he's examining the menu with such acute interest I wonder if perhaps I should recheck my own—clearly the secret to eternal youth, the cure for cancer, and the solution to ending world poverty is in the fine print at the bottom.

"I could catch the goddamn crab myself for nine dollars! Hell, I could catch a dozen crabs for half that price! I grew up crabbing, young man, and believe you me, this is a rip-off. Rip-off!!" He continues to look around for moral support, but everyone is embarrassed, awkward, and silent. "She'll have the regular steak," he snaps with a nod at me. Then shakes his head and rolls his eyes, muttering under his breath at my impertinence.

He orders the same for himself and another $18 glass of scotch.

I shrink into myself, totally humiliated. I'm an adult. A professional. The head of public relations for a 750-billion-dollar company—the very company that owns his company, by the way. I should be able to order my own goddamn nine-dollar crab special.

Then again…apparently not.

The next morning, I arise at the inhuman hour of 4:00 am, pack quickly (the complimentary toiletries are distinctly *not* worth bringing home), and rush to the lobby to wait for the SVP. After last night, I'll do anything to avoid seeming like the stereotypically high-maintenance female.

In the car ride back to La Guardia, my head bobs with exhaustion, but I won't rest even a moment. If the SVP can tough it out, I can too. I look out the window, and we fill the drive with silence. At 6:40 am we land back in Boston. Just in time to get to the office and start my day early.

Note to self: next job should not include travel.

"Yoginis," Thea says at the beginning of the next training weekend. "I have great news."

My imagination runs wild. *Famous yoga guest? Free lunch? Abbreviated training hours?*

"I've been meaning to tell you that I lost all your checks from the last few months."

I mentally calculate the cost of the immersion and subsequent workshops multiplied by 22 trainees...the total is over $66,000.

"...And I thought I was going to have to ask you all for new ones, but last night I found them in the pocket of my other jacket. Isn't that great?"

Yeah, *great.* She temporarily lost $66,000. Three thousand dollars of which was mine. Really confidence-boosting and professional.

Summer giggles quietly next to me. "It's like the universe is protecting me."

"What do you mean?" I ask.

"I haven't actually paid for any workshops. Thea and I just have an understanding that I'll pay her when I can, which is...well, I don't know."

This renders me speechless. I've never missed a payment for anything in my life. Paying your bills isn't *optional.*

"Conventional time boundaries and money...well, they're like...really toxic," Summer continues. "They could totally cloud my creativity. And I have to be like free in order to *create music*."

The idea of not paying for a workshop is unfathomable to me. I wouldn't even know how to ask for a one-week extension. But apparently not everyone suffers under such constraints.

Thea clears her throat, snapping my attention back to her. "So...this weekend we'll be taking a formal look into our own being. We'll analyze our own energetic defaults. Then we'll use this greater understanding to explore the healing potential of our yoga practices." After a pregnant pause and a pointed sip of tea, she goes on. "We should all consider ourselves *very* lucky because this is quite a luxury."

Leaving thoughts about finances behind, I try to ooze gratitude. But I don't feel grateful. Still desperately behind from the honeymoon and falling even further so with each unnecessary business trip, I've been working late every night to try to catch up. But it's a fruitless endeavor. It's as though I'm adrift in a leaking rowboat in the middle of the ocean. No matter how fast I bail water out, more and more pours in faster and faster. This creates the modern-day woman trifecta of doom: I feel out of control, overwhelmed, and exhausted. And, frankly, that makes me grumpy. And not in a cute seven-dwarf-y kind of way. More in the Darth-Vader-I'll-choke-a-bitch way.

Given that I remain in chronic arrears at work, I'd been sorely tempted to skip a month of yoga training and make it up next year. But I'm stubborn and determined to gut through anything in order to complete the training in a year. Plus, it was a well-known fact in the corporate world that only whiny little bitches who can't handle real life take time off.

Unfortunately, stubbornness and the refusal to see oneself as a whiny little bitch are the un-doers of modern-day sanity. So here I am, determined to take this workshop come hell or high water. But now my brain is refusing to settle in and focus on taking a formal look into my own being. How am I supposed to focus on *that* knowing that mountains of work are looming back at the office? And what's the relevance of this to becoming better at yoga? Not that we'd done any yoga so far in this training....

I try to quiet the judgmental, anxious thoughts racing around my brain with deep, calming breaths. I'm determined to tune in. I *will* make this work. *Even if,* and here I mentally grit my teeth, *I don't see the point.* Even if I might think this exploring thing is a big, stupid waste of time.

Summer begins peeling florets off a head of raw broccoli and eating them. Each crunching bite echoes loudly in the room. She stops long enough to ask if anyone has a pen she can borrow. Brinley sighs heavily and then, as though she'll take care of this because she *has* to, walks one over to her.

Thea resumes. "Okay guys, let's begin by exploring—or discovering!—our defaults. *Depressed* practitioners will approach their practice slowly, slumping, looking down, completely uninterested. *Anxious* practitioners will speed-race through *asanas*, constantly looking around at other students, judging their own practice and that of others, completely unmindful."

I'm guilty on every count of first-degree anxiety. I swallow hard and await punishment.

I'm not disappointed. She assigns us 30 minutes of practicing everything we're *not* supposed to do: our energetic defaults. I roll my eyes and rebelliously hope she sees it. We're smart enough to comprehend her point—our defaults are going to yield a cruddy practice. Do we actually have to *experience* the crud? I consider asking but know that I'll be universally shot down. Brinley or Jaznae would be only too thrilled to offer New-Age babble on the yogic epiphanies they intend to experience.

Resignedly, I whiz through my transitions, think about dinner, relive my most embarrassing moments, and stare unabashedly, even downright intrusively, at everyone around me. I catch Hazel and Jessica watching me as well, and we exchange guilty smiles. I'm basically one step away from reaching for a gossip magazine and cracking open a beer with a caffeine-sugar-non-vegetarian chaser.

In a shocking twist that nobody (nobody!) could've anticipated, the practice isn't a good one. I emerge even more anxious and agitated. Thea proved her point. I don't feel the need to talk about it.

Apparently, not everyone shares that inclination.

"*Sooo…?*" Thea prompts leadingly, with a small smile that looks more like a smirk.

"That was awful," Summer says. "I feel awful. Just *terrible.*"

This serves as a veritable starting gun for a yogic race to the bottom. A few others bemoan their similar effects, and the competitive nature of the class quickly takes over for who feels the worst. Thea nods knowingly after each admission as though to convey that, yes, yes, she knew it would be like this. It's all playing out exactly as she'd known it would—this is what comes from embodying old patterns.

"I couldn't stop thinking about the squirrel I ran over on the way here!" Gloria cries with great animation. She pauses and I try not to picture the flattened body and fluffy tail. "My entire practice was consumed by the stain of death. Nothing could be worse than that."

Brinley eyes her beadily. "I feel completely disassociated from my mental and emotional bodies. *That* is the worst possible thing anyone can feel. Especially for a *mother.*"

"I felt my inner essence connection shift from deeply authentic to disconnected," Jaznae chimes in.

"My mind-body connection is totally strained," Kim adds.

"My throat chakra feels blocked," Gloria says, massaging her throat.

Finally after everyone has confessed how absolutely dreadful, how very toxic, and inner-essence-eroding the practice was, Thea leads us through a counterbalancing restorative practice. Why we had to reinforce those negative patterns at all remains a mystery.

Once she deems us energetically balanced (although this didn't rebalance me), Thea launches into the importance of a focus on alignment and how it also aligns the mental and emotional "stuff" that people carry both on and off the mat. "In addition to our emotional patterns, we also have our movement *samskarras*—it's easier to just follow our patterns and go through the motions."

Guilty again, I wonder just how often I've done exactly that—gone through the motions on the mat, just punching the yoga time clock so to speak? Or done the same at the office, with colleagues, with friends, with family, even driving? Smile and nod and meanwhile my mind's a million miles away. I realize with certainty that I don't want to just "go through the motions." At all. Ever again.

"We like poses that we're good at," Thea continues mercilessly, truthfully, and I'm suddenly very interested in studying the floor. How many times have I requested or simply just jumped into my favorite poses—the ones I'm good at—instead of pushing myself to try and fail and try again the ones where I fall out, lose my balance, feel limited, unsuccessful, or just plain unable to freaking do it?

"But that only allows the practitioner to stay stuck in old patterns, stuck in their old emotional, mental, or physical 'stuff,' which may not be serving them positively. And that doesn't allow healthier patterns to emerge. Ask yourselves, what could emerge if we weren't so busy preventing it?"

The concepts of mental patterns and their physical expressions sift slowly into my brain. I think of Jessica, who is so flexible that she sits easily in full lotus, coiling her feet up onto her upper thighs. In fact, she'd sat happily thus entwined in the passenger seat on the way to Whole Foods earlier and I'd missed a green light as I stared over at her, amazed she could just zip into full lotus! In the car! Without even warming up first!

My tight-as-old-lady hips creak and resist when I attempt to do the same even after a vigorous, hip-opening sequence. But in class earlier this week, I'd noticed to my surprise (and darn it, hadn't Thea just said that looking around at others was something anxious people shouldn't be doing?) that Jessica wasn't as mobile in other poses. When we'd done hamstring lengthening poses, she'd been high up on blocks, looking uncomfortable and clearly counting the seconds until we were out, while I'd been able to cascade forward with comparative ease and wanted to stay for longer. And sure enough I hated doing hip-openers and she requested more, and she didn't enjoy hamstring poses and I gobbled them up. *We seek what we're good at, but we should do more of what we aren't,* I think nobly, feeling righteous for all of four seconds. But who has the discipline to actually do that? That's no fun. I'd avoid a class like that. I even avoid it in the classes I *do* take.

"The most important thing to remember is that there is a continuum of alignment based on people's bodies and their stuff," Thea continues.

Wait...*what?* If that's true, then there are no concepts of proper alignment, no improving poses toward a commonly agreed upon ideal. And my entire reason for taking this training—to refine and enhance, in essence to *perfect* my own practice—has been built on a foundation of incorrect assumptions.

As though she had not just turned my world upside down, in effect wiping out my entire reason for being here in the first place, Thea marches on to activation of the sympathetic and parasympathetic nervous systems.

I dutifully take notes, but I'm still stuck on the alignment issue. I feel crushed by the collapse of my idealized definition of what yoga is. Strangely, as I let this settle into my overstimulated brain, I also feel kind of relieved. Sure, the deflation of my expectations is disappointing, but it's also freeing. For years on the mat, I've struggled against my body, trying to twist and push and lengthen it in ways and poses it may never be able to do. And if I let myself get all squishy and metaphysical, maybe there's a correlation with the rest of my life as I struggle to cram myself into various things off the mat as well: the corporate mold, high heels, suits, working with people I don't respect, jobs I actively despise.

The consequence of being trapped for *years* (a decade?) in the limbo between what I want and what I actually do daily, between who I innately suspect I am and what I've tried to force myself to be instead, was the erosion of my sense of authenticity, a steady decline of respect for myself, a steadily increasing sense of frustration, and the ultimate decaying of creativity and hope. I wasn't happy, but lost and overcome with inertia, I felt powerless to do anything about it. And that was even more pathetic.

Yoga had provided me shelter from my own life for nearly as long as I'd been constructing the very dynamic from which I needed shelter. In its most-recent iteration, the Tri Dosha slow-flow practice with props that I'd begun when I'd applied for this program, created a sense of freedom and support that nourished me, bolstered me, and allowed me to emerge, renewed, to face my job again.

So maybe I'll never have Jessica's hip flexibility, but maybe that's okay because I'm still going to harvest the benefits of the poses, and within the continuum of my anatomy, I'll master them. And by "master," I now mean accept that I *won't* master them. My next question, conjured up by this monkey-chatter brain, is: How will that translate to my life *off* the mat?

"Today we'll continue the work of this weekend by attuning our gaze more deeply on healing." Thea's voice is wise, stoic, and knowing, but it doesn't stop me from wondering what the heck that means, why we're doing this, and what she wants us to heal anyway. In spite of the breakthrough that Thea's astute questions had led me to, I wasn't ready to delve into healing stuff.

"Yoginis, why are we doing this?" Thea asks as though reading my judgmental mind.

Wait. Can *she read my mind?* I wonder guiltily, looking down, then frantically tell myself, *Don't think about sex. Don't think about sex. Please do NOT think about sex!* Of course now I can think of nothing but sex. So then I change my plea to, *Please don't let Thea be psychic. Please, don't let Thea be psychic....*

Thea's eyes rest an extra beat on me. Then she continues. "Why? Because if we can heal ourselves, we can help heal others." She smiles, nodding eagerly at us. "We need to always remember the complete interconnectedness of the mind-body. If you work on the physical body, even if you only work on the *asana* class level, you can help heal—or conversely reinforce—negative patterns or experiences. In Tri Dosha Yoga, we believe each person holds the knowledge to create their own healing. We as teachers do not heal them—students heal themselves. When a student feels fully supported on every level of their being, *tremendous* healing can occur." She pauses for a well-timed sip of her herbal tea. "Awhile back, I told you I had a student who fractured her hand, remember? And how her doctor told her she'd have to have surgery?" Thea pauses again and there is complete silence. It's clear that everyone remembers, but it's just as clear they can't wait for the chance to relive it. "But I suggested she hold off and do some restorative yoga a few times a week instead. Sure enough, four weeks later, the fracture had healed on its own—*without* surgery. That's the sort of results that can be achieved when yoga is practiced therapeutically."

There is a responsorial wave of "oohs" and excited scribbling. My immediate response—*wow! That's so cool!*—is just as quickly silenced when I remember that I fractured my big toe a few years ago while running down a flight of stairs in high-heeled sandals (a move only true geniuses try). The doctors weren't sure if I'd need surgery or not because the break ran dangerously close to the joint. But the fracture had healed on its own—without surgery or restorative yoga—in about four weeks. Now, maybe I am a super-speedy healer (a necessary trait for high-heel-wearing geniuses), but from my limited understanding, depending on the type and severity of the break of course, it actually wasn't unusual for a fracture to heal itself in that time frame. Alas, I wasn't super-speedy, but only average.

So why was Thea presenting it as a small miracle? Or at least adding *some* sort of disclosure? Could it be because that wouldn't support her argument about yoga's "incredibly healing results"? Revealing only certain slices of the data reminds me of financial services…and not in a good way.

I don't have time to ponder it as Thea tells us she had a student with cancer who, during a class had seemed ready to release "something," and, at Thea's prompting, had breathed that "something" into Thea's hands. The next week the student's cancer markers started to decline.

Now there's nothing less than awestruck reverence around the room. Healing cancer? Knitting bones back together? Thea and the extraordinary possibilities she's revealing have merged into one glorious, shining beacon. Which alone presents an incongruity (one of several), as Thea's devoted so much time to emphasizing and reemphasizing the importance of not making yourself, as a teacher, the holder of "the magic." She's spent so much time on the importance of empowering students, how we should always remember that it's the *yoga* that does the work. But what about the incompatibility of now telling us about this student with cancer? What role was Thea suggesting she herself had played when she'd offered the student her hands and told her to "breathe it out?" Healer? Holder of the magic? And by telling this story to her trainees, wasn't she also creating a high—and some would say scientifically impossible—standard for us to follow? Or were we supposed to just admire it?

Issues with Thea's inconsistency about the role of a teacher aside, I also had to question her assertions about the role and power of yoga itself. With the introduction of "achieving incredibly healing results"—of having the ability, knowledge, and power to heal one's own body, Thea put some pretty intense stuff out there. On one hand, it's…well, tantalizing. To say the least. But what about those *incredible healing results?*

I'm torn between allowing myself to get swept up in the euphoric hopefulness that's swirling around the rest of the trainees—of course I, too, want to believe that anything is possible and in the curative power of the mind—and plain, ugly skepticism. Assuming the story was unwaveringly factual (and I had no reason to think it wasn't), *how* had this happened? Was it coincidence—the medical treatment the student was presumably pursuing outside of yoga simultaneously kicked into gear that week? Or did it fall into that category of the medically inexplicable but certainly true?

Beyond what I considered a healthy level of suspicion, I wasn't sure how I felt about the healing properties that Thea claimed yoga possessed. I also wasn't sure how I felt about Thea's choice to make these claims. Could I ever be comfortable retelling these stories? Would I even be comfortable being part of a *community* that retold these stories? And, on a wholly practical level, as a fairly compulsive hand washer, I couldn't stop wondering what Thea had done with the cancer after the student breathed it into her hands? Had she dropped it on one of the dirty blankets? Done some sort of ceremonial hand washing? Chanted?

Once again, I have to wonder: *Where* am *I?*

I'd filled out my application form a year ago, thinking that I was signing up to learn about alignment and perfecting technique. I'd come to advance my poses but had tumbled down a rabbit hole to an entirely unexpected world. I don't know what to do about that.

When I finally get home, bleary eyed, exhausted, and back aching from the damn floor, I find Thea's sent the homework out—early for once. In addition to the pages of questions, there's also a required update of my individual project, which I'm still working on in terms of "rewiring" my "neurological patterns." Translated into human-speak, that'd be reducing my chronic anxiety and subsequent insomnia. In hindsight, the whole urban yogini thing felt sort of like offering to paint the living room while the structural integrity of the house was rusting/rotting/molding.

But then, it was so much easier, so much *nicer*, to do the fun touch-up/decorating/finish work than to roll up my sleeves and dig in to the deep-down structural stuff.

Chapter Fourteen

The City that Never Sleeps…or Flushes

Introduction to Assisting, Welcome to Chaos

Work travel isn't letting up. I'm on the road every week—which I now know does not mean getting to explore cosmopolitan international cities, but does in fact mean eating a crappy road-food diet in between racing to meetings 14 hours a day while work piles up unrelentingly back at the office. Rounds of emails with my yoga group to try to set up a meeting are even more frustrating. Jaznae suggests meeting that night even though I've told her I'm traveling. I suggest the first weekend I'll be home, but that doesn't work for her. I suggest breaking into subgroups and reconvening later. Nobody responds.

My inability to sleep in ever-changing hotel rooms is a separate Goliath to be fought with tools like rage and Ambien. The cumulative effects of work travel are a fattened, acne-speckled, sleep-deprived lunatic. And this week, that lunatic's back in New York, for meetings with the advertising team, the branding committee, and the PR teams from two partner companies. I'm scheduled to go home on Friday afternoon, just in time to share my weekend with the yogis.

Until then, my temporary home is a hotel room, which, despite being upwards of $600 a night, may in fact be an establishment of questionable repute. Upon returning to my room after the first PR meeting, I find housekeeping had indeed visited my room…and in addition to the generic mini soaps, they'd also left a fecal log in the toilet that has to be at least ten inches long.

Duly impressed, I briefly consider immortalizing my discovery with a quick camera phone shot. Nunnally, at least, would appreciate this. We share the same juvenile sense of humor. I could even use my distinctly unfeminine ten-inch hand span for scale in the picture. But realizing this ploy would require closer physical proximity to a stranger's excrement, I quickly discard my initial photographic impulse.

Instead, I try to flush with the stylishly pointed toe of one shoe. But instead of flushing, the toilet floods—spouting from the bowl like a veritable fountain. Perched as I am, precariously on one foot with the other midair on the handle, I'm unable to retract my leg in time to avoid the surging water.

So yes, I get a stranger's poo-water on me. And that's never good. But because the water is literally gushing forth like a geyser, by the time I *am* able to scramble in an ungainly fashion out of there, the contaminated water is already about half an inch deep in the bathroom and rushing into the bedroom. I begin frantically running around, getting everything out of the way of the impending flood. I've never seen a toilet belch forth so much water at such a velocity. It's this germ-phobe's worst nightmare, live and actually happening.

Frantically, I call the front desk. "The toilet! It's flooding! Somebody…somebody…clogged it! Not me! I just got back! But you should hurry! The water's already coming out! And I need help with my stuff!" I'm torn between trying to defend myself and getting someone up here ASAP. But by the time a bellhop, accompanied by a plumber, arrives minutes later, the room is already flooded and water is pouring out into the hall.

Staying safely on the quickly shrinking dry portion of the carpet, I call after them, "Hey, guys? Listen. I just got back to my room and found the toilet was clogged. It wasn't me, I swear! I think it was housekeeping…." My voice trails off at their unmoved faces. "Um…do you think I could get a new room?"

"Lady, you gotta go talk to the front desk for that," the plumber snaps in between vicious thrusts with the plunger.

The bellhop is busily loading my bags onto his cart. He studiously avoids lobbing any accusatory looks my way. "Do you mind?" I ask, climbing on the cart like a gondolier and gesturing at my open-toe leather high heels. If I were in boots, or even closed-toe shoes, I'd slog through with him, but I'm not getting sewer water on my bare feet. "I'll hop off as soon as we're in the hallway."

After a large tip for the bellhop and a quick, but thoroughly embarrassing chat with the front desk rep, I walk into my new room with high hopes…and am met with what appears to be the set for the next episode of *Law and Order*. The stench of fried food, stale smoke, and dirty bodies assails me. The bed is unmade, the TV is blaring. Clothes and bedding are strewn all over. Just then the toilet flushes loudly. This one is clearly still occupied and practically roped off with police tape. I pivot on my heel and head back down to the front desk.

The third room I'm assigned has a suspicious large brown stain on the sheets, but I figure it's preferable to the poop and the crime scene, and I don't want to be the pain in the ass who keeps demanding to be moved. It's like sending your food back at the restaurant and risking the staff spitting on it.

I carefully arrange myself as far away from the bed stain as possible, commanding myself to sleep without moving. By strange coincidence, this toilet also spouts like a fountain, but I learn to flush and maneuver out of the way like a ninja. I wonder idly if these things only happen to me.

Hopes aren't high that the rest of the week will improve. The universe is clearing sending me a message: my life is shit.

"Welcome to the beginning of therapeutic yoga," Thea begins on Friday night, handing out mismatched workbooks. "Still paying that karmic debt," she adds with a laugh.

Brinley smiles and shakes her head as though that's the cutest thing she's ever heard.

"Before we start, I just want to remind everyone that we're nearly at the half-way point of our training."

Jaws drop, people groan, and there's a resounding chorus of "Noooo!"

Thea nods and smiles benevolently. "So…just a reminder to keep thinking about the *Seva* Rotation opportunity. And if you want to be considered, let me know in your study questions."

Back in the immersion, Thea had mentioned something about this—selecting three graduates to teach one-year rotations at studios that Thea partnered with in both Boston and southern New Hampshire. The studio charged only five dollars for the class, presumably to ensure there would be some attendance, and donated all the money to animal rescue. Let's be honest, if not for a discount and a good cause, why else would students want to subject themselves to what must inevitably be clumsy, first-time teaching at the hands of someone who's barely more than a student themselves?

The usual suspects straighten up a little taller. Eyes slide sideways, sizing up the competition. Energy crackles around the room. There is the undeniable air of a nose-flaring, hoof-stomping, equine-snorting out-of-my-way-or-I'll-mow-you-down race. But of course, it's carefully veiled under a yoga facade.

I lower my gaze and reach for my dark chocolate-covered snack bar. They can have it. I glance at the clock and wonder when we'll get a break and if I'll have time to go get a slice of pizza.

"This weekend, we'll take the inward-looking work we've done so far on ourselves and bring that clarity and compassion to students," Thea says, curtailing my mental chatter. "We'll work on this all weekend—and then we'll assist live clients at the end. Why is assisting important?" The question is rhetorical. "Because you can have a dialogue with a student's body and assist in their evolution. Because you can personalize a class. But remember: cranking a person into a pose doesn't help them, and in fact can seriously injure them. I've literally seen students leave other teachers' classes on stretchers."

The terrifying possibility of that hangs, unwanted, in the air. I swallow hard as a shiver of nervousness runs through me. The prospect of being the one on the stretcher is just as scary as being the one who caused someone else to be on a stretcher. I feel myself start to sweat.

Thea nods gravely before she continues. "*But* when we're trained and mindful, we can bring tremendous healing and awareness to students so they can access this growth *themselves*. Now, who'd like to share their concerns around assisting?"

Summer is crunching noisily on the entire length of a celery stalk. "I'm feeling totally insecure…like I'll never be any good," she says in between chomps.

"I guess I'm mostly concerned around boundaries. I'm not very good with boundaries. So I'm thinking about how I could end up bringing that into teaching or assisting," Gloria says, in her eager way.

"I guess I also fear judgment…like, 'oh, she sucks,'" Summer tacks on to her first admission.

Noemi, wearing the "Vagina!" T-shirt once again, talks about the importance of boundaries and the similar importance of maintaining them in her therapy work.

Brinley raises her hand. "I think we also need to be really mindful about protecting our own bodies—especially those of us who suffer from ligament and organ-related dysfunction." She places a hand on her abdomen. "Ever since The Birth of my daughter, I've been extra-mindful to protect my vulnerable abdomen."

Jaznae chimes in without bothering to raise her hand. "Aaactually, I'm feeling compleeetely confident in my ability to assist in a mindful way. I have no worries or concerns."

Again, that distinctive blend of musical trill and blustering confidence. I look over at Jessica and roll my eyes. She shakes her head. I should've found some excuse—any excuse—to migrate out of the group project with Jaznae.

Although I won't admit this to the class, in addition to the toe-curlingly terrifying possibility of injuring someone, I'm also really freaked out about getting other people's sweat on me. I know it's pathetic. I know I'm officially entering a tailspin of neuroses. I know I should be thinking enlightened yoga thoughts and willing to hurl my body over the landmine of whatever yoga travails students face like Victorian gents laid their capes over puddles for ladies. I should probably be willing to slather students' sweat all over me like tanning oil if it will help advance their practices. But instead, lowly non-yogi that I am, I just want to avoid the sweat—actually all bodily fluids—of strangers.

The idea of touching people I don't know, especially sweaty ones, is just too weird. Unless it's a code red, def-con five, national-security-breach-level emergency. And then, I'd like totally do it.

Thea sips her herbal tea and smiles. "Okay! Are we ready to see some assists?"

The rhetorical question has a predictable effect: a flurry of excited clapping as everyone gathers around her.

I only had time for one cup of coffee before class this morning. I'm not fully awake but am somehow faking it, propped up against the wall. A yawn escapes and I glance around guiltily.

"I'm going to demonstrate various assists. Who wants to volunteer as a student?" she asks.

Almost every hand in the room, except Jessica's and mine, jolts up as though the torsos connected to them have been zapped by electric cattle prods. Thea seems delighted. "Oh my. How will I ever choose?" she muses aloud. "Last year, nobody wanted to volunteer. I guess you just never know. " She shakes her head, laughing gently at her lovably unpredictable students. "Well, does anyone feel like they need help with a pose?"

Immediately, all the same hands shoots up again.

"I'll go," Brinley says, stepping forward decisively. "I think it will benefit the group to see a body with a serious, noncurable condition."

"Okay! Good!" Thea says perkily, ignoring Brinley's dour tone. "We'll start with downward-facing dog, *adho mukha savasana.*"

Brinley assumes the inverted "V" shape, pressing her palms and feet into the mat.

"Let's try the strap assist," Thea says.

Strap assist? I perk up.

Thea stands behind her and steps a leg between Brinley's legs. She loops the strap around the crease where Brinley's hips meet her thighs. With her hands on either side of Brinley's hips, Thea pulls strongly backward, toward her own hips. Brinley heaves a soul-deep sigh as though this is the most divine release of her life. I look for Jessica so I can validate the awesomeness of this moment and nearly collide with her.

"Yeah, I got that from a male assistant once and it was super weird. I hadn't seen him approach and so I guess I kind of tensed up. And then he pulled back on the strap and intoned in this super deep voice, 'Just breeeeaaathe.'"

As though we're 12, we convulse in giggles.

Thea shoots us a look. We immediately sober and straighten up.

And so it goes: Thea asks for volunteers and there is a cacophony of, "I'm bad!" "No! *I'm* bad!" "No, I'm the *worst*...the absolute most terrible." Then Thea picks someone, and they basically execute a perfect pose as they bask in the spotlight.

"Well I sure need help," Harper, the grad student from Tennessee says, when Thea calls warrior two. "I'm terrible."

"Okay then! Come on in!" Thea says, delighted.

Harper steps into the circle and slowly arranges herself into the pose. She faces us, her feet wide apart, her arms stretched straight out to the side. She turns her right foot out and bends her knee in a deep lunge. We all walk around her, watching, taking notes. Everything looks just about perfect. She looks strong, aligned, and warriorlike.

"I need two assistants," Thea says unexpectedly.

Brinley and Jaznae leap forward.

Thea has Brinley stand in front of Harper, Jaznae behind. Then she loops straps around Harper's upper thighs and has each assistant pull firmly in opposite directions for eight *ujjiy* breaths. Time slows to a crawl. The entire room waits and listens to Harper breathing.

"Now release," Thea says. The assistants let the straps go slack. She turns to Harper. "Breathe into surrender."

Brinley and Jaznae glide forward, their faces carefully arranged to convey the spiritual righteousness of having been honored to be a part of this rite of transformation. They remove the straps from Harper's legs.

Harper looks like someone just ran over her cat. Her eyes are red and brimming. She pauses for an endless second, then races from the room.

Jessica and I glance at each other in a mix of concern and confusion. *What in the name of Krishna just happened?*

Thea, as ever, isn't rattled. "Now, we'd never do that assist unless we had our own assistants—" She pauses as I consider that nobody here will have an assistant, let alone two. "And we knew the student very, *very* well. When we surrender into a pose, all sorts of things can get triggered." She takes a slow sip of her tea. "Okay, who'd like to volunteer next?"

If it's possible, all the usual hands shoot up with even more vigor.

On the last day of the workshop, Thea starts us off with a morning meditation on authenticity and serving others. The theme of service becomes more apparent as we prepare to assist our first real class. For the remainder of the training, Thea will hold a free class in the course of each workshop, which gives the community a fun little perk and gives us students to work with.

I'm more nervous than I thought was humanly possible. I can't believe we're actually going to be turned loose to handle real students. After the ominous student-on-stretcher story and innumerable hours spent sharing other horror stories about how we could physically maim and emotionally scar students, I've now worked myself into a state of analysis paralysis.

I was in an *ashtanga* class once, back in my overdoing, power yoga days, and the teacher stood on one woman's knees as she sat on the mat with the soles of her feet together, because the teacher was convinced the student's hips could open more. It's been years, but the woman's wince of fear and pain is still burned into my brain. Most horror stories come from similar overdoing, competitive, push-your-edge practices, not the gentle, safety-conscious schools of thought like this one. But in spite of this, and the countless hours we've spent on modifications and nondoing, I'm still scared. Even Harper's reaction the previous day was anxiety inducing. She's acting fine today, but I avoid looking at her anyway, if only to give her some privacy.

Thea leads us into the Great Hall—a room we've never been in before. It's cavernous—easily accommodating 80 to 100 people. "You would not believe how crowded these classes get, so don't let any latecomers in," she cautions.

Now I'm even more nervous. I slink to the back and try doing anti-anxiety breathwork—putting my individual project into action—as I brace myself for the stampeding herds. The door opens and students file in.

All ten of them.

Unfortunately, there are 22 of us trainees, so assistants outnumber students more than two to one. This foments immediate chaos. Compound this with the fact that most of my fellow trainees cannot wait to get their eager little mitts on some real, live clients—with the notable exception of Jessica, who is firmly in my anxiety boat, clutching an oar, ready to row—and the situation quickly ratchets up to bedlam on the heels of pandemonium. I step back and watch as the trainees circle the students like buzzards. They wait for the smallest misstep so that they can swoop in and demonstrate every single assist we learned, intermittently looking over to Thea, hungry for her approval.

I forget the breathwork as the class progresses and the level of competition intensifies—both for the chance to make an assist and for Thea's elusive approval. Overeager trainees repeatedly elbow and shove me out of the way as they hone in for the kill...uh, I mean opportunity to execute an adjustment.

Little do they know, I'm utilizing my finely tuned corporate skills to stay out of the way and do nothing, yet appear fully engaged and totally busy. I don't seek Thea's approval and I'm not ready to touch strangers, but when she catches my eye and points to the center of the room in a "get in there!" way, I jump guiltily and follow orders. My presence in the melee is wholly unnecessary as trainees continue swarming about. The current bobbles me around. I wander aimlessly.

By sheer coincidence, I happen to be accidentally loitering, trying to look busy, next to a student who eventually needs a shoulder adjustment. I look left and right: no one. Panic sets in. I'd better just do it. I take a deep breath and reach out toward her. Immediately, Kim and Jaznae, rushing from opposite sides, smoosh me, sandwich style. I disentangle myself and step back as the two grapple over who gets to do it.

It's the final straw. I spend the rest of the class on the sidelines, trying to appear involved, but not really wanting to be. I sidle off toward Jessica at the back corner. She's combing through her hair. At least I'm not alone in my reticence. I carefully avoid Thea's disapproving gaze at my nonparticipation..

After the class ends, we reconvene. "Thoughts?" Thea asks.

Immediately, at least 15 hands shoot up.

Thea looks over the group wisely; nods approvingly.

"It was amazing." Brinley says. "My own journeys—both of motherhood since The Birth and my own physical healing," she clutches her abdomen, "lent me such compassion with assisting."

Another approving nod from Thea opens the flood gates.

"Yes—eet was *magical*!" Jaznae chimes in.

"It all came together!"

"I felt so useful!"

"I feel like I changed their practices!"

"I witnessed evolution!"

"I saw latent parts reactivate and new neurological patterns develop. It was so powerful." This was from Kim, the blond psychologist who seemed to be developing an incurable thirst for Thea's approval.

"*Deeply* powerful," Janet echoes, and I wonder if the thirst for approval is contagious.

"It was so much harder than it looks. You make it all look so effortless, Thea! This really just helped me appreciate the amazing teacher that you are," Summer adds.

I look around incredulously. Um…excuse me, but what the hell is going on? Had I fallen asleep? Was this a dream? Had I slipped through a crack in the space-time continuum and fallen into an alternate reality? (And why, as an aside, do I sporadically worry about this theoretical possibility?) Had these people just been in the same class I was in? Maybe I'm over my BS quota—both literally and figuratively given the recent toilet-clogging incident—but this is just a little too much for me to swallow. I raise my hand tentatively.

Thea's gaze zeroes in on me, the green light to speak.

"Um…." I'm nervous, but determined. "I guess I'm just wondering if I was in another class or something," I attempt to diffuse them with humor, which falls flat, "because I had a totally different experience. I thought it was chaotic, competitive, and totally out of control. I felt like people were competing to do assists and racing each other to get to the students. I kept getting shoved out of the way…." My voice trails off.

Thea looks at me. There is silence in the room, disapproval in the air. "Is chaos a negative thing for you?" she finally asks.

Isn't chaos a negative thing for everyone? I wonder, but the way she asks, the fact that she has a PhD in psychology, and the fact that I'm in a roomful of people who seem to be the opposite of everything I am, makes me doubt myself. Even if it *were* a negative thing for every single person here, nobody would risk Thea's disapproval and actually admit it. "I…I guess so." I stutter, reddening further.

"Like, if I said there was going to be this crazy chaotic street party, would you think that sounded fun?"

"No," I admit, now concerned that I'm the un-fun party-pooper in the group.

"You need to look at chaos and your relationship to it. Think about that," Thea says.

I have the uncomfortable feeling that I'm being psychoanalyzed instead of heard.

The class regards me smugly. There's a room-wide vibe of, *"Ah, mystery solved. Sara has chaos issues."* Picking up on Thea's lead, there is a rush of disagreement with me.

"I wasn't getting that at all, Thea." Kim says. "I felt like we all worked together very fluidly and smoothly."

Jaznae hurries to make herself heard. "I felt *fully* supported by the group and my fellow trainees, and the mindful boundaries I'd set for myself at the beginning of the class."

I stare at her dubiously, wondering if she thinks she'll get bonus points for using the yoga SAT words, "mindful" and "boundaries." Had she forgotten basically hip-checking me out of the way when I tried to make an assist?

"I get what Sara is saying," Jessica pipes up. "I got elbowed by a few people who wanted to make assists on someone standing in front of me."

"Well, I don't know where *you* were standing, Jessica, but it all felt very *sattvic* to me," Brinley admonishes sternly.

Thea awards her a nod.

"Very *sattvic*," Kim agrees, earning another nod from Thea.

"I just found myself wherever I happened to be," Summer says randomly, to nobody in particular, as she munches on some sort of unidentifiable cruciferous snack.

"Okay. Well, I think there was a lot for us to learn here today if we were willing to see it," Thea says and closes the conversation by reminding the class that group projects are due next training.

A tinge of panic sweeps in. I suddenly realize that my group never responded to my follow-up email suggesting alternate meeting dates or splitting into subgroups. Now, with less than a month to go, I'd need to be even more diligent.

I do a few rounds of anxiety-lowering breathwork and feel slightly calmer. Our "project" was about as straightforward as you can get: it was one blank page that you could use to write out your teaching sequences. In far less time, with far more at stake, I'd pulled together complex presentations for press conferences. In comparison, this was so *not* a big deal.

We break for lunch and Jessica, Hazel, and I bolt for the door. "Lunch?" I call to Janet, hoping I can talk to her about our project.

She nods and joins our procession. We're intercepted, however, by a skinny white guy coming in with an adorable, dark-skinned African American toddler. They make a stark contrast. He scans the group and waves at Brinley.

Brinley sashays over. She pecks him on the lips and reaches for the baby. "Everyone, this is my partner and our daughter, Persephone!"

There is a coo of fluttering as everyone gathers to admire the beautiful baby. Summer looks around like she's the guest of honor at a surprise party, trying to figure out how this all could've happened. "Wait…is she adopted?" Summer asks, verbalizing the question we're all thinking.

Brinley snorts. "Yes."

Janet, miraculously unfazed, continues toward the door. "Lunch, guys?" she calls toward our group.

Brinley catches Janet's arm as she walks past. "Janet, now that I have a black daughter of my own, I just want you to know that I understand your *struggle*. I *get* it."

Janet, Jessica, Hazel, and I stare, agape, at the lily-white Brinley and her equally white partner. They are suddenly the whitest people I have ever seen. Their very whiteness is blinding.

Janet sets her jaw and says nothing.

"You know, your *struggle*." Brinley continues in a lowered, confidential voice, pointedly excluding Jessica, Hazel, and me. "The trials of being African-American can really only be understood by those of us who actually experience them firsthand." She shifts the baby to her other hip and continues. "You know, I was grocery shopping last night with Persephone, and some woman actually had the audacity to come over to me and say 'What a beautiful baby—your husband must have really dark skin.' I mean, *really*. Can you believe that such racism still exists? I tell you, it's so hard raising black children. But of course, we're so blessed to welcome the opportunity of this beautiful challenge into our lives."

"Yeah," Janet says slowly, "growing up under segregation and having spent my whole life as a black woman, married to a very dark-skinned black man, and having raised two now full-grown black children, I can definitely tell you: it's not always easy to *be* black or to raise black kids."

With that, she pivots on her heel and walks out. Hurriedly, Jessica, Hazel, and I follow.

When we're finally settled and chowing down, Janet rolls her eyes. "I just *knew* she'd have a black baby. I just knew it. As soon as I realized that she hadn't actually given birth, in spite of her many references to "The Birth," I just knew she'd have to go out and adopt a black baby. *I just knew it*."

I'm impressed at her keen skills of detection. "Wait—*how* did you know, though?"

Janet rolls her eyes, gives me a look. "Honey, trust me, you just *know*. That woman *had* to have a black baby."

Chapter Fifteen
A Bush Grows in Boston: A Poem

Yogis Not Being Yogic

Vomiting Vicky and I are back on the road—San Diego this time, to meet up with Charles and some of the sales guys. On the flight, Vicky plunks down in first class while I plod into the bowels of coach and squeeze into a middle seat. No sooner are we airborne than a frazzled flight attendant traipses up and down the aisle, frantically calling my name until I self-consciously flag her down. "Your *boss* sent this with her compliments," she snaps, shoving a vodka nip and a can of tonic at me. "Boy, she's a piece of work, huh?"

"You can only imagine," I confide. "Actually, you probably can't and don't want to."

We arrive about six hours later to meet the senior management of a newly acquired company. Our mission is to provide them with PR, marketing, and sales support. We are quickly hard at it—corporate style, over spreadsheets and catered mini-muffins—all morning until it's time to get to know one another over lunchtime icebreakers and a fatty, unpalatable buffet.

The consultant who's been hired to "synergize strategic expectations" between Investorcap and the new acquisition announces that we're each to get up and share, in under 30 seconds, our proudest moment.

My eyes roll into my forehead. I repress a groan.

The Meat, here to represent the sales team, strides to the front and assumes an appropriately wide stance. "Beers with the Red Sox in Miami! Yeah! High fives! All around, guys, all around. High fives for The Meat."

Rotely, the rest of the group talks about medals won, honors earned, marathons run, and sales goals met. It's a blandscape of the usual accomplishments.

Until it's Vicky's turn. "I've just composed a poem as I've been sitting here. It's about my passion for growing bonsais." She clears her throat loudly, glances around to make sure everyone's listening, and reads off her well-inked napkin. "The growth within me…and the growth of my bonsai. Only a drop of rain, only a kernel of dirt, yet growing…growing…like me, pruning you, my tiny bush, keeps you small…and yet…you are…free to grow…grow and grow. Oh life, sweet, sweet life. How you grow. How you know. How you are. What I am." She bows her head, ending the soliloquy and retakes her seat at our table.

There is stunned corporate silence. Even the consultant looks unsure. The Meat, at least, looks impressed at the mention of a tiny bush. I glance at Charles. He's studying his shoes as though his life depends on it, the picture of mortification belying rage.

Vicky sits back down, takes up her cutlery, and saws away determinedly at some sort of protein covered in white gravy. "So, do you guys ever like to smell bad things?" she asks nobody in particular. "You know, things that kind of stink, but really smell good?"

Again silence. Endless, awkward silence. The hysterical urge to giggle rises up. I cough into my napkin.

Thea opens the weekend with a chant in Sanskrit. To my surprise, this is starting to feel commonplace.

"First, an announcement. Laura," she gestures to a new woman sitting a few feet behind her, "is our assistant for this weekend. This commences a new assistantship program where graduates of this training can apply to work as my assistants for future workshops. Start to think about whether this might be a good fit for you. It's unpaid, of course, and I can't cover meals or transportation, but it's a good opportunity to get experience working with me."

Immediately, there is excited room-wide scribbling. I have a feeling Thea will have more assistant applications than she'll know what to do with.

"So…why do we assist?" Thea asks.

"We" refresh "our" memories as to why, which basically means that Thea issues broad prompts, and the usual suspects—led by Brinley, Jaznae, and Kim—are only too excited, too thrilled, too *utterly delighted* to expound on these clues, their hands spasmodically jerking up like jack-in-the-boxes on crack. Of course, it's inadequate to just look at their notes and spit it out. No, as usual it's all *mirror, mirror on the wall, who's the most yogic of us all?* as they compete to demonstrate not only their mental knowledge of the material, but also their understanding to the core of their essential inner selves. This means spouting back Thea's definitions, infused with their own organic analogies culled from their inner awareness of their fundamental essence with words like "chakra" and "moonbeam" intermittently thrown in.

After lecturing about an hour, Thea pauses. "Let's take some time so we can sit and absorb the effects of the morning. Then we can journal about our latest insights."

A heavy silence pervades the room as the yoganess oozes from every pore and trainees eagerly flip open their yoga-themed, Sanskrit-embroidered journals with an air of: *I have so many yogic insights emanating from my inner essence, I'm mentally reaching enlightenment as we speak.*

The quiet is suddenly disrupted by Summer noisily opening a paper bag. The crackling is almost deafening in the still room. Heads swivel disapprovingly toward her, as she sets about messily spreading cream cheese on a bagel, though more seems to end up on the floor. Mesmerized, I watch her scoop it up and lick it off her finger, then repeat this several times. Finger swipe the floor, up to the mouth, lick it off, and back to floor, blissfully unaware of the many sweaty bare feet that have trod that very spot.

Brinley pauses from her extensive journaling to look over at Summer. If possible, she straightens just a bit more. "I haven't eaten dairy since I started practicing *ahimsa.*" At Summer's blank look, Brinley clarifies, "The yoga principle of *nonviolence to self and others.* Are you aware that dairy cows are forced to be in a permanent state of lactation in order to continually produce milk? Have you thought about the fact that when you eat…that *stuff*, you're actually breast-feeding from a *cow*? How would *you* like to be forced to be into a permanent state of lactation?"

Summer freezes mid-chewing, still holding her bagel up to her mouth. She looks unsure what to do next: continue eating her cream cheese bagel, which only exists because of enslaved bovine breast-milk-making, or stop eating, spit it out, go hungry and dairy-less. Brinley lifts her chin righteously and looks away. Summer eventually unfreezes and keeps eating.

Naturally, I can respect people making the choice to be vegan, but Brinley's holier-than-OM routine irritates me and has from the first day. *Just another day in yogaland,* I tell myself.

At the end of the evening, Thea announces that project presentations are due Sunday, and I realize with sudden dread that I still haven't heard back from anyone in my group. Between work and travel, the group project had slipped through the cracks and completely off my radar.

I actually feel sick. I've never missed a deadline or turned in a project late in my entire life. As a geeky, obsessive, type-A overachiever, I graduated *summa cum laude* from college, number one in my department. I'm the sort who volunteers for *extra* work—not skips out on the *original* work.

I try to catch my group members, but they've already left. I call Kim as I drive home. For some reason, her cell is the only number I have. The yogis communicate only by email. Kim groggily informs me that she's already asleep. I apologize and tell her I'll catch her tomorrow.

The next day, we resume the "practice and demonstrate poses" exercise from the previous night.

Anxiously, I wait for the next break so I can approach my group. When Thea finally grants us five minutes, I notice that my group members are all seated together at the other end of the room. Everyone else is sitting at Thea's feet, but my group is in a tight, exclusive huddle. I walk over, all of a sudden feeling that something is very wrong.

"Hi, guys!" I chirp, determined to seem positive. "I just wanted to touch base about the project. I wanted to see what I could do in advance of the presentation. I was thinking I could offer my graphic design skills? Or I could do some complementary materials...I know it's kind of late, but I figure since it's only one page, it's not a huge deal. I can definitely get whatever needs to be done, done." I see their stony faces and my voice trails off uncertainly.

"Yes, Sara," Jaznae says in her showy, majestic way. "We have removed you from our group as you were not contributing at the level the rest of us were. So you are no longer a part of this group." With her hands, she makes an encompassing gesture around the rest of them and a shoving gesture toward me, palms out.

I stare at her hard, gloating face, not understanding. "Sooooo..." she draws it out. "*Thaaat* is *thaaat*."

"But wait. Hold on," I finally manage, my brain scrambling toward logic. "I offered my thoughts on the form, same as we all did. So I *have* contributed. I'm sorry I missed the meeting and scheduling's been hard—but I was on my honeymoon and since then I've been traveling for work. I sent you guys the idea about sub-groups and the dates that I *could* be there and nobody ever responded...."

"We had another meeting this week."

I look straight at Janet. She won't meet my gaze. "So didn't it occur to you guys to...I don't know...get together when I could be there? When we could all be there?"

They aren't moved. "We did email you, but we never heard back," Kim says sternly. "So we did some processing...."

Jaznae cuts in. "And we decided that you're out." Her tone, triumphant and hard, brooks no argument.

I look down. It's just plain humiliating to sit here, arguing what is clearly a losing battle. I'm desperate, but I won't beg. People are starting to stare. I accept defeat resignedly. I've been kicked out of my group—a group I never wanted to be in. By one of the rudest, most ridiculous people I have ever met in my entire life. *Wow. Total low.* "Well, if that's how you feel…I'll figure something else out." I hope I sound steadier than I feel as I get up and walk shakily over to Thea. I can't believe this is happening.

"We think that would be best. *Namaste*," Jaznae calls after me, and then they bend into their huddle and start whispering.

Yes, I think sarcastically. *Namaste. The divinity in you honors the divinity in me. Absolutely.*

"Um…Thea? My group just told me I've been kicked out," I say, smarting with the shame of being rejected, but somehow also feeling like it's my fault.

Thea nods, face placid. "They told me last night."

I freeze. *Thea knew before I did?* The question of why any of them didn't try to talk to me directly hovers at the edge of my mind, but at this point I just want to triage the situation and move on.

Thea leans back and plants her palms on the floor behind her hips, extending her legs out in front of her. She seems remarkably unconcerned by this development. "I'm not sure what's going on, but at this point, I guess you should try to form a subgroup with someone and get another project going."

Fine. That seems easy enough. I remind myself once again that it's a one-page yoga project for Pete's sake—not a dissertation for a PhD in rocket science.

Still, it's the embarrassment of being evicted from the group in the first place— a deep scalding sense of disgrace that whatever the group and the circumstances, I'm not wanted. The fact that it's a rag-tag bunch of yoga students at a teacher training doesn't really matter. Rejection and exclusion cut just as deeply on the playground in fifth grade as they do in the adult sphere.

I nod, biting the inside of my cheek—hard—in an effort not to cry. I'm not sure when I picked up this technique, but it works. *I will not cry. I will not cry. I will not freaking cry.* I don't allow myself to cry at work and, come hell or high water, I will not cry at yoga. It's freaking *yoga*, after all! I expect cliques and backstabbing at work, but I wasn't braced for it here. Here is where I let my guard *down*. It's supposed to be a bastion of peace—a sanctuary of serenity. My escape.

Instead, it's the opposite. I've been kicked out of my group—the leader of which is a wannabe "ahteest," yoga teacher trainee who seems hell-bent on creating drama at every turn. Kim's and Janet's involvement is more unexpected and therefore upsetting. Janet—my restorative partner, lunch buddy, and fellow victim of Jaznae's rant about college? Kim—a *psychologist*? I just had not seen this coming.

I take a deep breath and kick into survival gear. Mission: get through this. Tactic: whatever it takes. Technique: appear unaffected. I won't let them see I'm upset.

But I *am* upset. I'm hurt and embarrassed, and still fighting the tears burning the backs of my eyes. What cuts the deepest is that I'd let my guard down here— *here,* where I'd had to reveal my deepest scar. And it was supposed to be a safe and caring environment because it's *yoga.* Under the guidance of a world-renowned teacher of teachers. With a PhD in psychology.

As I'm waging this internal war, the world-renowned teacher of teachers has meanwhile ordered everyone to pair up for a blindfold practice to train us to lessen our dependence on sight. Because I was delayed by the group expulsion and subsequent ruminations, I find myself partnered with Gloria, the only other person wandering around helplessly looking for a partner.

"Sara! Hi!" she says in her warm, eager way.

I manage a wan smile for her, appreciative of her welcome, but just wanting to get the heck out of here. *Please, no word vomit today.* She invites me onto her mat and, reluctantly, I tie her scarf around my head to cover my eyes, then begin feeling for her alignment as Thea leads the class. I can't concentrate on anything other than what just happened.

As I fumble around her shoulders, it hits me that I'm tired. Really tired. On a bone-deep, broken-down, weary-ass, old-lady level. I just can't keep up this pace, working at the intensity this job demands, traveling all the time, always sleeping in a different hotel, waking up in the dark, startled and not knowing where I am, eating crappy food, never getting enough sleep let alone a second for myself, coming here once or twice a month for endless, emotionally draining, mentally taxing, physically exhausting days…and then trying to maintain my marriage, my friendships, and my family relationships in the in-between moments. I can't keep pretending that I'm on top of everything. I should just admit it: *I'm totally depleted. Body, mind, and soul.*

Assisting solely through touch, deprived of sight, is too much to ask right now, and I feel hot tears slide rebelliously down my cheeks under Gloria's scratchy wool scarf. I sniffle mutinously, and command myself to stop—*no sniveling, dammit!*—as I continue groping Gloria like some sort of overeager teenager in the backseat of Dad's Buick.

It's over 85 degrees in the studio and I'm sweating through my hair under the scarf. Between the heat, the scratchiness, and the bitter taste of rejection and self-pity, I get progressively more irritated until I rip the scarf off my head and throw it churlishly on the floor. Startled, Gloria twists up to look at me, taking in the tears. Her noticing only upsets me more—can't I just have one *freaking* moment of privacy?

"Isn't this amazing?" Her voice is full of wonder.

I stare at her. *What the* hell *is she talking about?*

"The blindfold is so powerful! It's okay, though. Stuff comes up when you do a blindfold practice. Close your eyes and allow your evolution to happen. Give birth to yourself."

I'm literally at a loss for words. I try desperately not to snap, "What the *hell* are you talking about? This whole thing sucks the sweat off hairy ass!" Instead, I manage to say, "I'm sorry. I need a break. I'll be right back."

"It's okay!" she says eagerly. "This is really powerful! You should just let it happen!"

Immediately, Laura, the workshop assistant, is at my side. "Do you need a break? I'll take over."

Her kindness shatters me. If she had ignored me, I might have made it. I might have made it all the way to the car where I could have hidden the shame of my weakness, and nobody except Gloria would ever have known. And she'd probably attribute it to the magic of the blindfold—an alibi that was fine with me.

Why is it that kindness, the one thing we most need at low moments, is also the undoing of us—sneaking in to penetrate our carefully constructed defenses and shattering the face we so vigilantly present to the outside world?

As it is, I nod and run to the bathroom where I slide down the wall, press my face into my hands, and dissolve in tears. This whole situation, and my intense reaction to it, is totally unexpected. I never cry. I've dealt with far worse at work. Hasn't my hide been toughened to the approximate consistency of rhinoceros skin at the hands of Vicky and the female predecessors before her? Those crazy corporate bitches will chew you up and eat you for their carb-free lunch if you're not guarding against it—out-maneuvering, out-strategizing, out-playing them every second. But I hadn't been prepared to play those games here.

And, besides, I really hate those games. My goal was to get away from all that. But it seems that even here, in my yoga refuge, that was not to be.

Having snuck in my cell phone—contraband on training weekends—I call Nunnally and relate the events.

"What?!" he exclaims, protective and outraged. "That's crazy! Who the hell *are* these people? It's a freaking yoga project! This is high school bullshit. You shouldn't have to deal with this and you especially shouldn't be paying hundreds of dollars to have to deal with this. Come home."

As usual, just hearing his wonderful, beloved voice soothes me as I feel his protection shining through. Buoyed up and innately stubborn, I decide to finish the evening out.

Laura, Thea's kindly assistant, knocks. "Hey, just wanted to let you know we're done if you want to come back. But...are you okay?" she asks through the door.

I open the door and summon a smile. I hope my eyes aren't red. "Yup! Fine!"

She touches my forearm. "It's a lot, I know. I always tell people it's great to do the training when you don't have anything else going on in your life. You know? Like I waited until my kids went off to college and life was quiet."

"I wish my life were quieter." I choke out a bitter laugh that's more of a hiccuppy sob. I've never wanted a quiet life more.

Back in the studio, we reconvene in a circle and Thea assigns us a reflection journaling exercise.

Petulantly, I refuse to sit in the stupid circle, choosing, instead, to sit by myself, leaning against the wall. I can't even attempt writing in the aftermath of the ousting.

"Sara? Are you joining the circle?" Thea asks, pointedly ignoring my chosen seat. Every head in the room swivels in my direction.

"No, thanks. I'm good here." I try to keep my voice even.

Brinley scowls disapprovingly. Jaznae does her best to look noble.

"Are you sure you don't want to join us?" Thea presses.

"Yeah," I pause, yoga-style. "I want to sit here tonight."

Thea frowns and turns away. Her disapproval is as tangible as the smell of sweaty feet. In unison, the trainees follow suit, and I'm forgotten, left in the dust with my aberrant ways.

Thea leads a closing chant focused on *ahimsa*—kindness— to self and others. Jaznae's voice, ironically and discordantly, rises above all the others.

Posers, I think bitterly as the closing note is still hanging in the air. I leap up and leave the building as though my hair is on fire. I cannot get home fast enough.

Nunnally is waiting at the door, arms open, lower lip protruding in the sympathetic faux pout that always makes me laugh. I drop my yoga bag and cry tired, snotty tears into his shoulder nook. My entire body is filled with dread at the idea of having to go back there. At one am, after compulsively making Nunnally dissect and analyze the whole bloody thing from every conceivable angle, I finally decide to skip the rest of the weekend. I've paid for it, after all, I can choose not to attend if I want to. I email Thea my decision.

Nunnally promises me brunch the next day to cheer me up. Easily plied with food, I accept. I guzzle two glasses of wine, the deep red *rioja* warm and relaxing, and plummet into a numb sleep.

When I wake up ten hours later, I still have a deep sense of dread in the pit of my stomach. I drag myself to the computer and get a thoughtful, well-worded response from Thea about why I *should* come to the training. She assures me that group project presentations will be put off until the following month regardless. I shudder at the idea of further confrontation. Thankfully, I've already slept through the morning session.

Jessica texts me that afternoon to check on me. I respond that I'm fine and will fill her in on my absence later. She immediately writes: "Nice work skipping out on assisting the sweaty, unwashed volunteer masses. Jeez, even in Maine, we have signs: 'please be considerate and shower before you arrive.'"

Back at work on Monday morning, I get a very unexpected email from WS Brinley, expressing how saddened she was to learn of my decision to leave the training program and asking me to reconsider. She offers her support of my "situation."

Humbled by her kindness, I immediately feel guilty for how mentally harsh I was to her about her wandering spleen. I'm a jerk. *But wait...who said anything about leaving the program? I have absolutely no intention of quitting halfway through!*

I call Jessica and fill her in on being voted off the yoga island. She sighs loudly. "First of all, you did the right thing. And you didn't miss anything. After we assisted the class, Thea said she needed to talk to us and basically said that she's noticed that our class is *seriously* lacking support and kindness and that one of 'us' was missing—because she didn't feel welcome."

Immediately, I'm ashamed, as though this is all somehow my fault. I can't get past the thought that by admitting hurt, I've shown weakness. Has the corporate world taught me nothing? Never show any weakness! Ever!

"So then your group got really defensive and started arguing with Thea, and Janet started crying and said she didn't know what to do, and Jaznae and Kim were trying to tell Thea that it was all *your* fault. And Thea was telling them, 'It's not about fault, we're talking about a pervasive unkindness in this whole group.' And then the whole class got into it and Gloria said that Thea sets 'a container of unkindness' and that trickles down to everyone else. And this went on and on and on. I just sat there. I could see it wasn't going anywhere."

I'm suddenly very, *very* glad that I didn't attend.

For the first time in my entire life, I'd ignored my inner mantra of *must finish every single, tiny thing* and had actually tried to give intelligent thought to what was good for me, a novel and liberating concept. And even if that only translated to missing one day of a yoga workshop, it still felt pretty radical to a goody two-shoes like me.

And then, suddenly, it's the holidays. I wear my best little black dress and favorite red heels to Nunnally's firm's party at a bar downtown, where I smile and nod and make polite chit-chat with his co-workers while trying to subtly work into conversations with partners just how dedicated Nunnally is to his job.

In turn, Nunnally wears his best black suit to the Investorcap holiday party, held at a swanky hotel. As we walk in to the high-ceilinged ballroom, bedecked with gilt-coated chandeliers, I retrieve our seating cards and head slowly through the crowd toward our table. My heart sinks; already seated at the table is Charles and his wife, some SVPs, and...Vicky. Next to her is a handsome but nervous-looking guy. I wonder how she's managed to dig up a real, live date.

"Hi everyone!" I say, nervously wondering where to sit.

Vicky downs the rest of her champagne and slams the glass down with unnecessary force. "We're off to dance!" she says by way of greeting, grabbing the dark haired guy's hand and towing him away.

"The Patriots are looking strong!" Charles says to Nunnally, nodding at the chair next to him—the ultimate honor. Jealous glances from around the room slide our way. Nunnally, unaware, falls into a seemingly effortless conversation about football and I lapse into silence, proud that Nunnally can speak this macho language so fluently and, by association, earn bonus points for me.

The band starts to play a slow song and Charles's wife, petite and perfectly coiffed, nudges his arm. He reluctantly lets her guide him to standing. "A bit of marriage advice for you," he leans in to tell Nunnally, "Keep the little lady happy. Happy wife, happy *life*, fella."

"Shall we?" Nunnally asks, standing, after they're gone. "Gotta keep the little lady happy."

"Shhh!" I hiss, laughing, in case anyone overhears his mocking tone.

"I'm obviously kidding. We're a power couple." My heart flutters; power couple sounds pretty cool.

On the dance floor, Nunnally twirls me in toward him and we sway to the music. "Wow. You're a good date," I say, smiling up at him.

He's about to respond when, in my peripheral vision, I see Vicky approaching, *sans*-date. "Cutting in!" she coos, ramming her size-zero frame between Nunnally and me. Without any other choice, I step back and she tango-stomps him to the opposite side of the dance floor. Face burning, I shuffle my way to the edge of the floor, trying to play it off that this is totally cool and I *like* dancing alone to a slow song.

From the sidelines, I watch Vicky dragging Nunnally around. Other couples step back to watch the display. I catch sight of her date heading toward the bar.

A song later, Nunnally manages to disentangle himself from her clutches. "Wow," he says under his breath, as we head back to the safety of our table. There,

Charles having fulfilled the obligatory "happy wife" dance requirement is waiting to continue talking sports with Nunnally.

I sip my champagne and surreptitiously survey the room. The Meat is staked out at the bar, talking to an admin in a green sequin mini. Everyone else is heading toward the buffet. At the far end of the room, I see Vicky's date, half-carrying her out, her head slumped on his shoulder. And so it is…another day at Investorcap.

Nunnally and I spend Christmas with his family. To my own shame, I haven't been home for a holiday in a few years…but it's just so much easier to flop with Nunnally's nearby family than to pay the inflated rates and battle hordes of grumpy, stressed travelers all the way down to Philly to be with my aunt and extended family. This is compounded by the increase in work travel. If I don't have to be on the road for Investorcap, I just want to be home.

I invite Annie and Hanna to join us at my new in-law's house. I look across the table at them, comforted to have my sisters present in this unfamiliar family gathering. Guiltily, I realize that I haven't seen my sisters since the wedding. I drink the rest of my red wine (ignoring my now-standard guilt over not abiding by the yoga rules) and set a new year's resolution to make more time for them. Yes, work is intense and it feels like I have yoga trainings every weekend, but especially now that they live in Boston, I need to make time to see them. I miss them.

I shake off the unwelcome thought that I need some time for myself as well and that, although it was originally supposed to be my refuge, I now need some time away from the training. I shudder and make myself focus. My second resolution is to not think about yoga training or Vicky until after the holidays. I'm determined to stick to it.

Chapter Sixteen
Where the Ka-Chiggity Is

Yoga and the Spine: Backs Aren't the Only Thing
Out of Line

On the first Monday of the new year, I return to the office to find a gift from Vicky on my chair. Vicky herself is still on vacation. Inside the plain brown paper is a canvas tote stamped with, "Proud Supporter of the American Bonsai Club." I know it's rude to look a gift horse in the mouth, but this looks suspiciously like a free gift after donation.

Betsy steps into my office and clears her throat. She's holding up a sweater that's roughly the size of a couch. Approximately 32 Betsys could fit in it. "My holiday present from Captain Theatrical—is this a subtle hint I need to lose some weight?"

Angela joins us. She holds up a Bonsai Club key chain. "At least you can return yours," she says, nodding at Betsy.

Betsy shakes her head. "Nope—no tags."

The Meat pops his head in the door. "Ladies," he drawls, eyeing each of us. "So...a little holiday gift action going on?" he says in that way of his that makes everything sound vaguely dirty. "Nice. Niiiiiice. Whatcha got for The Meat?" He laughs to let us know he's kidding. Kind of.

I dangle my newly acquired bonsai bag from one fingertip, but, shockingly, he ignores the free gift. "So...did Santa make it down *your* chimney?" I say, somewhere between mimicking him and attempting to converse in male financial patois.

The Meat gives no indication that he's aware of my sarcasm or the ridiculousness of being offered a bag that was clearly re-gifted to me. "Indeed he did, ladies, *indeed he did*. And I'm talking about inside the office too, if you know what I mean." He raises his eyebrows suggestively to indicate that the office rumor that one of the admins got fantastically drunk at the party and was alleged to have been found on The Meat's office floor, naked and waiting for him, is, indeed, true. I try desperately to void my mind of this image.

"And…check this out," he continues, reaching into the pocket of his infamous pleat-front pants and pulling out a monogrammed silver money clip. In its jaws is a wad of hundreds. "Nice, huh? Yeah, I ended up going for the man clasp. You know, the wallet was just getting too big with all the hundos….You guys ever feel like you have too much money? Yeah. Sometimes you've just gotta burn some of that cash."

He pauses, totally serious. Angela, Betsy, and I stare at him incredulously.

In a rare moment of awareness, he picks up on our incredulity and laughs. "Man, you girls gotta get over to sales. Sales is where the ka-chiggity is. I mean…sure, the company's trying to stiff me on a $50k commission from last year, but I say, 'Please, I find that much between my couch cushions.' You gotta think big picture if you wanna be a winner." He stretches his arms over head and yawns languorously. "Think about it," he adds with a wink-double point at me. Then he saunters off toward Walsh's office.

Betsy shakes her head. "Social tundra, I'm telling you, *social tundra*."

My phone rings. "It's Vicky!" I say, recognizing her number. "But I thought she was still on vacation."

"Oh, she is," Betsy says. "She's probably calling you because I'm not at my desk. It's sad actually, but I don't think she has anyone else to call."

I take that in as I answer, "Hi, Vicky. How are you?"

"I'm fabulous! The weather here is absolutely fabulous and I'm having a completely fabulous time!"

"That's great," I say as Betsy whispers "I told you so!" and leaves with Angela. I turn my attention back to Vicky, who is launching into every "fabulous" detail of her vacation. I should probably be amused by the fairytale she's working hard to create, or maybe annoyed at the waste of time, but my heart feels hollow at the thought of having to call her employees because she has absolutely no one else to call, and I suddenly feel very, very sad for her.

The next teacher training workshop looms this weekend. As I emerge from the holiday hullabaloo and clear the cobwebs from my brain, I wincingly remember how my group ousted me, and, worse, that the ensuing turmoil was never resolved.

And now I'll have to face my group, and, gulp, *partner* with them to see rounds of clients who are coming in for free therapeutic sessions. This is even more terrifying than assisting the free community classes because we'll be working with them one-on-one in semi-private sessions *and* they have serious spinal issues and injuries.

Especially in light of this, the intrapersonal crap has to be resolved. It would've been ideal if any of the offending group members had apologized…or at the very least, dashed off the ever-chic faux-pology, "I'm sorry *you* felt upset. Let me explain where *I* was coming from…." But of course, that hadn't happened. I hadn't expected any better from Jaznae. But, frankly, I had expected a little more from Kim, as a psychologist, and Janet, as my buddy.

But the bottom line was they hadn't. So I figured that left me with two options: either ignore them (which, given the upcoming work, would be challenging), or somehow smooth it over enough so that we can try to concentrate on learning. Oh yeah, and there was also that small matter of trying to actually help the clients.

Then it dawns on me: Why am I dealing with this on my own when I'm paying thousands of dollars to train under someone with a doctoral degree in psychology and 20 years of experience in the field? Shouldn't she know a thing or two about conflict resolution? Knowing that managers appreciate employees who take the initiative, I email Thea about my plan to resolve the awkwardness of having been kicked out of the group.

"We've all been losing sleep over this but after the fallout last month, the entire group is ready to emphasize togetherness, unity, and the embracing of others' differences," Thea responds.

There's a scene in *When Harry Met Sally*, which I'll unabashedly state is one of the greatest movies ever made (and I will go to the mat over that), where Sally stares indignantly at Harry and demands, "Is one of us supposed to be a *dog* in this scenario?" That movie moment flashes into my mind now. Or in yoga speak, "Is one of us supposed to be the one with 'differences' in this scenario?" Sort of like one of "us" needs to examine her relationship to chaos?

And aside from that cryptic statement, call me a cynic, but I figure the chances that my group is suddenly ready to "emphasize togetherness and unity" are approximately slim to none. And Slim just left the yoga studio.

I take a deep breath and, between meetings and deadlines at work, pound out several drafts of a conciliatory email to Kim and Janet. I intentionally leave Jaznae off, because, let's be honest—I'm trying to make this work, but I'm not a miracle worker. Some kinds of crazy can't be fixed. I finally hone a version I'm comfortable with—one that walks the fine line between explanation and pointing fingers, blame and reason. And, in an effort to seem like a "real" yogi, I close with my fervent hope that we can "all move forward in a mindful, yogic way, following the *ahimsa* that we always meditate on, and that the new year will bring us closer to our inner divine, more-evolved selves." For good measure, I even add a smiley face—ignoring my cringing inner corporate editor—and send it off.

Which basically, translates to: I'm bending over backward to try to make this work. You could even say I'm in full freaking wheel pose trying to make this work.

Within an hour, I get a chilly response from Kim saying that if we are going to discuss the group, the *whole* group, including Jaznae, needs to be included.

Which I guess would've been fine if Jaznae had exhibited even one tiny semblance of sanity over the duration of the training. But, even more concerning, I sense from her choice of words that Kim, who I'd originally allowed off the hook as a mere accomplice to Jaznae, has taken a rather belligerent and inflammatory tone. She doesn't indicate that she wants to move forward, or that she is trying to be "yogic" in any way, or even that's she's one teeny, tiny bit sorry. The email feels instead like she's trying to start a fight and draw battle lines—all of them versus me. Before I can respond, however, a new email—this one from Jaznae—pops up suggesting that the whole group meet to clear the air.

I'm confused. I'd purposely only emailed Janet and Kim. So how did Jaznae get pulled into this? I scroll down and see that Kim forwarded my original olive branch message and her own chilly response to Jaznae and Janet, but had taken me off the chain so that they could discuss it amongst themselves.

But when Jaznae responded to Kim, suggesting we all meet as a group to "clear the air," she'd added me so that she actually was speaking to the "whole group."

I can't decide if this seems surprisingly mature and inclusive of her or whether it's a control issue—since she kicked me out, she figures she'll hang around and pick the meat off the carcass.

Almost instantaneously, yet another email pops up, another one from Kim. The first line reads:

"I am SO sick of this whole bullshit with Sara."

My stomach lurches as I realize this email is a botched "reply all" in response to Jaznae's message. Kim, not realizing Jaznae had added me to the string, had intended for this message to go only to Jaznae and Janet. The guilty embarrassment of eavesdropping and hearing something bad about yourself sweeps over me. I wish I hadn't seen this, and I know with a deep-down certainty that nothing good will come from reading the rest, but of course I read on.

I feel like her and all her issues have gotten in the way of MY training…. Now all of a sudden, HER ISSUES somehow become my responsibility to deal with. I'm not interested, that is why I was not warm…. I don't know her and don't feel obligated toward her….I'm sick of this victim act she's putting on. We three have a nice connection that has been tainted by this issue….I look forward to having more girls' dinners at my house and enjoying each other's company (without her!!!!!)

As I read, my yoga mentality goes out the window and I get progressively more pissed. Why is she blaming everything on me? When have I ever made myself out to be the victim? When have I gotten in the way of her (or, frankly, anyone's) training? Unlike the majority of the class who seem to be there for group therapy, I approach the training with professional discipline: I come in, do my work, and leave.

I read and reread the email. I contemplate trying to pretend I never saw it. But the idea of attending the workshop in the face of her outright hostility makes my stomach clench. Every cell in my body wants to run away. I'm simultaneously outraged by the hypocrisy of her attacks. So this time I don't hesitate. And I don't try to meditate under a Bodhi tree and deal with it on my own. I immediately forward the whole chain to Thea.

Thea responds surprisingly quickly for someone who, until recently, I'd thought might not know how to use a computer at all. She writes that she's sorry to hear about this, but I shouldn't let it bug me. She assures me that this won't be a problem this weekend, as the rest of the group is now "sensitized" to the issue of togetherness. She does, however, want to meet with my group members after the training tonight. She signs off, "DON'T WORRY!" and a lower-case "t."

Oh, but tiny t, I am *worried.* I hate confrontation and dread fighting of any kind. Ridiculously, I actually find myself feeling kind of afraid of Jaznae and Kim—as though I'm a little girl again and they're the scary playground bullies.

I think of my Uncle Martin's advice when I was trying not to get pulled into office politics in my first job. "Just walk away. Don't let 'em get you down, kid," he'd said amiably. "Never let the bastards see you sweat." The second part he'd also offered with equal applicability when I'd gotten laid off from my first job and had promptly driven, in tears, to his house for Chinese take-out and career advice.

I hope that Thea's doctorate and decades of experience outweigh her "we're all sensitized to the issue of togetherness" naïveté. Because from my jaded, cynical, corporate-whore experience, I know that that sort of thinking is indeed naive.

I pick up Hazel on the way to the training. She patiently listens, and, as is her way, says little on the lengthy drive as I compulsively obsess about what the meeting with Thea will hold.

"I wouldn't worry too much," she says calmly.

"That's what Nunnally said too," I tell her, as I proceed to ignore both pieces of advice "But I *am* worried." In fact, my brain is tightly clenched around this nugget of worry. I can do nothing *but* worry.

As I walk into the training, I see Brinley filling her water bottle. "Hey, Brinley!" I say, walking over. "Thanks so much for reaching out after the last workshop—"

She cuts me off. "Oh. Hello," she says formally as she brushes by.

I stare after her.

Resigning myself to never understanding the mystery that is that woman, I go to gather the requisite props for surviving a night of floor-sitting. I place myself a careful distance from Jaznae, Kim, and Janet—or at least as far away as I can be, given that we're in a circle. I try not to look at any of them or peek to see if they're looking at me.

I needn't have bothered. They're deep in a debate with Brinley about who should get to set up Thea's spot for her and who should fetch her props.

The class seems small. Several students I never really got to know are missing. Summer, wandering around distractedly and munching on something strange, asks if anyone knows where they are. Brinley, emerging victorious from the Thea-prop-fetching debate, states, "They have some *issues* to deal with and dropped out. *If* we're doing the work that Thea lays out for us, a lot of stuff can come up."

So this is it. Our first casualties. It could've been me. But it wasn't. I strengthen my resolve: I will not quit. No matter what.

Noemi sits next to me. Jessica, running late, nabs a spot near the door just as Thea arrives toting a boxful of what I can only assume are workbooks containing some sort of copying error. She drops the box on the floor and perches in lotus. Brin-ley sits directly to her right, close enough that only an amped-up Chihuahua in full-body lube would dream of trying to wedge its way between them, but far enough to convey the respect owed to a guru. Which is to say, not in Thea's lap.

Thea opens with a chant for *ahimsa*, community and appreciation. Of course, I can only focus on the irony, given my current situation. Well, on the irony and on trying to ignore my new yoga enemies, of course.

Thea opens her eyes. "This weekend is about embracing uniqueness. Break into partners and tell each other two things that you appreciate about them that are totally unique."

I turn to Noemi. "The first thing I appreciated about you was your unique self-expression through dressing and accessories," I tell her. "Like your Vagina! shirt from the first day of the training."

She laughs, shaking her head, mildly self-conscious. "Really? I don't remember!"

I almost burst out laughing. How can she not remember a T-shirt that says "Vagina!"?

I'm embarrassed when it's her turn to appreciate me. "Sara, there is such a gen-uineness of presence in you—an authenticity about you—a courage...and hones-ty...a vulnerability when you ask questions or challenge things in class. When you admit that you don't understand or even agree."

Now I'm the one who's surprised. I've felt so self-conscious all this time, sure that my questions only revealed that I don't belong. I'd thought I was annoying Thea and the rest of the class. Now Noemi, who I haven't even gotten the chance to really befriend, is telling me she appreciates this about me? *Really?*

"Really?" I say out loud.

She smiles and nods. "Really. Plus, you were the first person to come up and introduce yourself at the immersion. You offered me restaurant recommendations and made me feel welcome."

It's funny what memory yields. I'd sat next to her because she seemed friendly. Beyond that, I only remember the Vagina! T-shirt.

Thea rings a pair of chimes and the room goes silent. "Remember, when you're dealing with clients, especially those who feel 'different' or 'abnormal,' they may create stories around their conditions. Be sympathetic, but not indulgent. Honor the person's current experience and then help them into a new experience. And always hold on to the possibility that the story can change."

The simplicity of her words belies the difficulty of the concept. I write it down, then sit for a moment and try to let myself absorb it. You know, on some deep yoga level.

It occurs to me that this could be useful both on and off the mat. How many situations in both my personal and professional lives could this be applied to? *Understand the other person's pain or reason or story, but don't indulge it. Honor the experiences of others but don't get caught up in them. Always allow yourself to believe that their "story" can change.* It's basically a blueprint for navigating life and relationships.

I sigh. Despite her blatant naïveté, her blissful (or perhaps willful) ignorance of the bullshit that is daily life, and her annoying inability to firmly put an end to the cattiness that pervades this group, Thea can still make me stand still and question a previously unconsidered assumption.

I thought she should create, for instance, an environment that simply did not tolerate bullshit through her own leadership. But is she, instead, trying to create an environment that changes said bullshit? And given my small-group expulsion experience, I had to wonder if her theory worked. *Can people change? On the mat? Off the mat? Fundamentally?*

Somehow I get through the next two hours and Thea dismisses everyone. Everyone, except my group members.

We sit in a mini-circle in one corner while the rest of the class files out of the studio, casting curious stares at our group. When the last yogini has left, a heavy silence blankets the room. I stare at the floor as though my life depends on it.

Seeming perfectly comfortable, or perhaps deeply grounded in yoga-ness, Thea begins. "Sara reached out to some of you to try and resolve the lingering issues. That seems to have sparked a chain of emails…one of which originated from you, Kim, and which Sara was accidentally copied on. This was forwarded to me."

She stares directly at Kim, and I realize once again what an impenetrable force to be reckoned with Thea is. Though diminutive in stature, there is that sense of stern authority that I'd noticed from the beginning. She may *look* like a cross between a fairy and a ballerina, but she *seems* like a cross between Jackie Chan and the Incredible Hulk. I assume this has something to do with her being a therapist.

If I were Kim, I honestly might shit in my yoga pants.

Instead, Kim looks completely and utterly unperturbed. "Yeaaaah. Sorry about that," she says. She sounds anything but.

I suddenly remember Kim is also a therapist. *What's with all these tough-ass therapists? Am I the only one cowering here?*

Thea meets her gaze steadily. "This stops *here* and this stops *now*." The way she says it brooks no argument. "I've consulted the Yoga Alliance and they've advised that I'm within my rights to expel you. You need to know that whatever issues you have are yours to confront. Maybe you should consider taking a break for a few months to sort those issues out." She looks around at the rest of us. "That is, of course, an option for all of you."

I can't bear to meet her gaze. I can only think, *Please don't kick me out of your training! It would be too humiliating! What would I tell everyone?* Then, *don't be ridiculous. Why would I get kicked out? Rein it in, DiVello.*

Thea takes a breath, then goes on. "However, it is my hope that you'll *all* stay in the training and work to move forward." She stresses the word *all* and looks directly at Kim. "I think you have a unique opportunity to really work through some stuff here. Remember that challenge is always an opportunity for growth…an opportunity to emerge with a sense of healing and togetherness, compassion for each other, and nourishment for the self. I think that's what we should focus on here—the positives." She is smiling eagerly, wanting us to take that step.

I wish she would toe the line of being tougher. Ultimately, that's what these people were going to respect.

"Does anyone have anything to say before we close this chapter for good?"

Predictably, Jaznae speaks up. "Yes. I would like to address Sara with the group present."

Thea nods her consent. My stomach clenches.

"If there were actions of which I was a part that somehow upset and seemed unkind to Sara, then I would like to say that I'm aware of such part," Jaznae talks her way around in a grand circle, sounding still-regal and not even a little bit sorry.

I blink. If there was an apology in there, I missed it.

"Anyone else?" Thea asks.

I surprise myself by raising my hand. I clear my throat, anxious but determined. "You know, I just want to say that we've all had to make ourselves really vulnerable to each another, sharing stuff like our greatest scar, from early on. I let my guard down because this seemed like a safe place to do that and frankly, because we had to. So, I think it's really important that we continue to be aware of that vulnerability and to treat each other with kindness and respect. That's all I ask for."

"There *will* be respect," Thea says firmly. "This journey can be sweet and fruitful if we allow our labors to ripen to that point. I'm here to help you all on that journey. So let's move forward. See you tomorrow. Okay? Okay."

We all nod. For the first time, I feel supported by Thea. Could she have done more? Yes. But at least she did this much. It's a good feeling.

I keep my eyes down, careful not to look at anyone as I make a beeline outside. I'm afraid one of them is going to try to corner me away from whatever authority Thea represents, and then the shiz-natch will really go down. Like old-school meet-me-by-the-flagpole-and-I'll-kick-your-ass style.

Quickly, I collect Hazel, who I'd promised to take home. As we pull away, I see Jaznae, Janet, and Kim standing in a tight huddle across the street. I wonder what they're saying and feel the tight anxiety of exclusion once again.

I exhale for the first time in half an hour and turn to Hazel. "Holy crap. That was intense."

I wait for her to ask what happened.

She doesn't ask. She seems, as usual, completely unworried. "Eh, it'll be fine."

Hazel may be the most relaxed person I've ever met. If we were dogs, she'd be the canine equivalent of a basset hound in his 80s (in dog years, obviously); I'd be the energetic counterpart of a Jack Russell puppy who'd been stuck in a crate all day and was just *thrilled* to be out.

The irony is that basset hounds are my favorite dogs.

Hazel turns toward the window. She continues gazing into the darkness, completely at ease. "Just remember that you're in this training for yourself, no one else. And you're not responsible for how anyone else feels."

I try to slow my racing heart. I try to take calming breaths. I know if I don't dial it down to some sort of approximation of Hazel's level, I'm probably not going to make it into my dog years, let alone be able to sleep tonight. I wonder what it's like to be basset-like, level and steady, to not let events swirl you up in the center of their hurricane.

"Honestly, Sara, judging from some of the conversations I've had with Kim, it sounds like she's having a hard time dealing with Thea in general. She's using your project as an outlet for her frustration. You can't let it bother you." Hazel's voice is level, steady, uncommitted. She might as well be discussing the evening weather forecast ("Maybe it'll rain, maybe not. Either way, it'll be fine.").

It catches me off guard to learn that Hazel talks to Kim. Doesn't she know that Kim is sheer, unadulterated, blond evil?! And if they're such good friends, maybe *Kim* should give her a ride home. I mentally slap myself for these childish, vindictive thoughts. "But it does bother me," I insist. "First of all because I hate confrontation, and, second, because this whole thing became such a tangled web of issues when it never needed to be anything at all."

Hazel's still looking out the window, seemingly perfectly content. I wait for a response. And wait. And wait. I want to say, "*Hello*?" I'm tempted to check her pulse.

Her silence, her unwillingness to dissect and examine, to analyze and discuss this issue down to its very marrow—and then from several more angles just for good measure—are foreign and bizarre to me. If I were with Leigh, Jessica, or any number of my friends, they'd be providing all sorts of possibilities, thoughts, and opinions. They'd roll up their sleeves and leap into the fray with me. Hazel's silence is indeed foreign, but as it stretches on, it provides me time to reflect. It's kind of like being in the car by myself, except with companionship.

I use the silence to think of Thea's "hold on to the possibility that the story can change" proposition. Given our meeting, and both Jaznae and Kim's completely un-apologetic responses, was Thea still hoping that their "stories" could change? If so, that premise now seemed to be teetering precariously on the brink of ignorance. *Will-ful ignorance*. Or maybe just naive hope.

But at what point is it advisable to renounce ignorance or hope, and instead in-stitute action—even if that meant ending the situation in a crushingly decisive auto-cratic manner? A business—at least the business of this yoga teacher training—wasn't a democracy anyway. Thea was a leader, and an autocratic leader at that when it came to, say, crushing any challenges to her theories. I flash back to how she'd ended my challenging of the "magical" first assisting experience with a swift comment about me needing to examine my relationship to chaos. Questions about the merits of this philosophy aside, being a leader meant you should act like one all the time. Even if you didn't want to. And, over the past months, I'd begun to think that sometimes Thea *didn't* want to. The problem being, you can't just be a leader *sometimes*.

I can't help but think of my office, where my bosses seem to be weak yet auto-cratic leaders, where posturing, backstabbing, and bullshit are as much a part of the culture as cubicles and coffee.

It's incredibly disappointing to learn that this yoga world is just like any other workplace or group—it has its own share of bullshit and backstabbing. It's especially disheartening given that I'd come here seeking an escape from corporate life. I had idealized the yoga world into a gentle utopia of girl-power, support, camaraderie, and understanding simply by nature of it being yoga. I had drunk the yogic Kool-Aid in eager, glugging gulps.

Because this was a place of nonconformity where everyone seemed to be high on the sweet scent of progressivism and the universal acceptance of all lifestyles, orientations, choices, and expressions, I had wrongly assumed that it was also inherently a place of universal kindness and respect. The long fall to reality from that assumption yields a painful landing: yoga teachers—and yoga teacher wannabes—for all their New-Age talk about compassion and acceptance can really be just as messed up and bitchy as the corporate barracudas I work with. The only difference was that I *expected* it from the ones in suits.

I feel disillusioned.

Conversely, it's also strangely freeing.

I had spent the training thus far feeling that *they* were "yogic" and *I* wasn't. I had worried that their alternativeness, their lack of concern for personal hygiene, their I-don't-care-how-I-look-I'm-beyond-all-that-now vibe, and their self-help, pop-psychology idioms somehow made them innately "yoga people." While I, a non-vegetarian straight shooter who shaved her legs, and lived *and worked* in the city, somehow innately wasn't.

Now, however, I could see that some of my fellow yoginis were posers—wolves in yoga clothing—while others were just completely and utterly out to lunch. But they definitely weren't any more yogic than I was. In fact, as Noemi had pointed out, my "authenticity," my honesty in admitting that I didn't agree, that I wasn't experiencing a powerful inner transformation every single day of the training, was in fact more "yogic" than their empty claims to be embodying all that is yogic while going behind my back and talking smack, or kicking me out of the group without first taking two seconds to check in with me.

Until now, I had felt like I was on the outside of the training looking in. But starting now, I'm going to take a seat at the table—or in the yoga circle if you will. I'm as much an integral part of this group—as much of a "yogini," whatever that is—as anyone else here. From now on, I will worry less about what others think. I will throw self-consciousness to the wind. I will be bold and ask even *more* questions, be even more *honest*, call even *more* things out on the old smelly-foot carpet.

181

For the rest of the weekend, whenever we chant—to open, to close, to refresh us in between groups of clients, when the moon is in the seventh house and aligned with Jupiter—I make my voice heard. For the first time, I don't worry about how it sounds.

We see five rounds of clients each day, each with six to ten students in it, and all with various issues—scoliosis, sacroiliac joint dysfunction, kyphosis, lordosis, etc. We sit behind Thea in a semicircle and observe as she conducts intakes with each person to learn about their history of injury, then we pair off in two-person teams to serve as assistants for each client as Thea leads the semi-private therapeutic sessions. I make sure I don't end up with Kim, Janet, or Jaznae.

I try not to look around at anyone else, but I can't help but notice that Kim is going a little above and beyond with her assists. I roll my eyes and turn away.

In all, we'll see between 60 and 100 clients, each with a plethora of ailments, each requiring an exhausting amount of mental energy to think about the ramifications of the ailment, how to individually modify poses for them, how to prop their bodies, if there are contraindications, poses we can't use, risk to the client, how this is affecting them, and stuff that it's bringing up for them emotionally, all back to back without a break. Before you can process that, you're on to the group, trying to give them the same undivided individual attention.

Of course, every session runs late, eliminating our breaks and lunchtime. Groups of people back up in the hall as they wait for their timeslot, and we, brains overflowing and physically weary from lifting blankets, bolsters, and bodies, move like glassy-eyed yo-bots into the next session. Because to be a true yogi means having no awareness of time or schedules or punctuality or efficiency.

Chapter Seventeen
Almonds: It's What's for Dinner

Nun's New Yoga Habit

Vicky sticks her head in my office. "Eating again?" she asks, scowling.

I freeze under her glare, then deliberately resume eating my midafternoon snack of almonds and dried cranberries. "Yup. It's my snack time."

She edges inside and gestures to my small pile of almonds. "That's your *snack*? That's what I eat for dinner." She tosses a stack of folders on my desk and I fleetingly wish I was devouring a giant ice cream sundae instead. "I need you to look these over before tomorrow," she snaps, then licks her lips nervously. "Seeing those almonds is really making me hungry."

"Would you like some?" I offer, nudging the bag toward her.

In her trademark nervous tic, she smooths her skirt over her hips as though to check that the bones still protrude, that there is no trace of fat. "No." She hesitates another moment. "Well...maybe. But only five. But then that's five less for dinner." Carefully, she counts them out and shoves them in her mouth in one ravenous bite. "I just can't believe all you're eating," she adds, heading for the door. "So...*gluttonous*."

The Meat saunters past. "Ladies..."

"Well, hello there," Vicky purrs, simultaneously letting her glasses slip down her nose and gazing at him over them as she touches his upper arm. "How are *you*?"

The Meat pauses as he wrestles visibly between his need for female attention of any kind and his obvious desire to avoid the crazy redhead. The need for attention wins out. He reenacts the male "adjust" that he usually saves for meetings. "Doing great, Vicky, doing great," he murmurs leaning a palm on the wall behind her. "And how're things over here in marketing land?"

Vicky pulls my door firmly shut. Even so, I hear her forced flirtatious laughter. I focus firmly on my screen.

Charles is sending me to Beaver Creek, Colorado, to represent the business at a marketing summit at the Bachelor Gulch Ritz Carlton. Vomiting Vicky's not going. I'm too relieved to ask why.

I've never quite gotten the hang of these summits. As in, I don't really understand why I'm sent to attend them aside from the fact that if I'm not, there seems to be a lot of fear that other people representing their related businesses could get away with something. Or maybe take over something. Or maybe vote us out. So I go, and sometimes Vicky goes, and I take notes and make sure everyone sees and feels my mighty presence so they know they can't get away with anything or take over anything or vote us out of anything. Or at least that's why I think I'm there. It seems like a lot of wasted time and travel for what could be condensed into a two-hour conference call. But who am I to question spending tens of thousands of dollars to go and "summit"?

If I was a skier, I would've known that this is quite a desirable place to go. As I'm not a skier, valuing my intact body and wishing to avoid grievous injury and/or death, "Bachelor Gulch" sounds like a Wild West gold-rush sort of town where the deer and the antelope play, and seldom is heard a discouraging word and the skies are not cloudy all day. The reality, I learn upon arrival, is that it's been made to look like a rustic lodge, but is, in fact, the height of luxury at every step. My room, complete with a fireplace and mountain view, has Bulgari products...definitely worth taking home.

Somewhere along the corporate yellow brick road, I'd learned to judge the caliber of a hotel in part by the quality of its bathroom products. If it's generic, nameless, or labeled "soap," there's cause for concern. This will probably be matched by torn, stained, worn carpets, chipped and scratched furniture, towels that could be used as industrial abrasives to buff the rust off any surface, and questionable sanitation throughout.

The Ritz at Bachelor Gulch is at the opposite end of the spectrum: impeccably clean. Flawless service. Incredible care applied to each and every detail. Even the ultra-deep bathtub in my room is equipped with Bulgari tea sachets to soak in. This is the sort of place, I learn later that night, that if you don't finish your $24 glass of wine at the bar (yup, still a right-hand column orderer as well as a yoga rule-breaker), without asking, they happily pour it into a paper cup for you to take with you on your motorized sleigh ride up the mountain to one of Colorado's best steak-houses.

"Sweet! The Meat loves steak," The Meat, having flown in for the sales portion of the summit informs everyone. "Gotta fuel up before I hit the slopes."

For The Meat and the rest of the skiers, there are attendants outside the heavy wood-framed doors who remove your shoes and place your feet into ski boots, which they also fasten for you before they help you over to the lift. Ever swift on the up-take, it suddenly occurs to me why my ski-obsessed co-workers might have insisted on this date and location.

While I am in the Rocky Mountains, Nunnally, meanwhile, is in London for his own business trip. London is five hours ahead of Boston and Denver is two hours behind, so we're constantly calculating the time difference and trying to find stolen moments to talk between my all-day-long meetings and business dinners and his similar professional commitments. The outcome of which is, there is no time, and we don't talk at all.

"No worries, we can catch up this weekend," I text him.

"Sorry, sweetie. Flying to Delaware Friday to prep for a hearing Monday. But I'm off all next weekend," he texts back seven hours later.

"Can't. I have yoga training," I reply, despondent. Suddenly being a power couple isn't so cool. In fact, it sucks.

Day two of the summit includes an advertising committee brainstorming session—or, more accurately, brain-*numbing* session. Our ad agency is on a mission to discover what makes Investorcap the best. They need a nugget they can develop into something really spiffy that we can then tout to our consumers. But as nervous throat-clearing stretches into silence, the inescapable truth that we really aren't so great takes form as the proverbial elephant in the room. Yet another nondescript conference room, that is. It was impossible to ignore, but nobody wanted to be the first to say it.

As always, I'm drowning in the mental tedium that spirals into desperate thoughts of dry-erase-sniffing rampages, but, on this particular day, the unique blend of mental tedium and escalating levels of being fed up drives me to desperate measures of a different sort. I take a deep breath and say, "Let's just be honest: we're not the best. We aren't the best company and we don't have the best products."

Utter, petrified silence greets this admission. Adrenaline sings in my ears. My cheeks burn. The room starts to spin. I don't know if I'm having a panic attack, a total meltdown, or am about to faint. This is the greatest moment of my professional career, with the possible exception of Vicky's tiny bush soliloquy and subsequent stinky smell admission. I've never felt more vitally alive. Or terrified.

The silence stretches and euphoria fades into panic. I'm sure to be drowned in a sea of robotic disagreement. I'll be unemployed and homeless after all.

"Sara's right. We're not market leaders." Someone from our West Coast office bravely seconds me. And it's like opening the floodgates and soon everyone acknowledges these truths: we aren't the best in any way. We don't even have the best people. There's absolutely *nothing* special about Investorcap.

I freeze, delighted and delirious. *Is this really happening?* What a relief to drop the curtain of pretense, in a conference room behind locked doors obviously, and speak the truth.

In the midst of my euphoria, I see the moment of panic in our ad agency rep's eyes and I can practically read his thoughts, *How the hell am I going to sell this company?!*

"Why do you all work here then?" he finally asks.

Drunk on the enormous relief and ensuing high of honesty, I want to shout, "I have no freaking clue! To pay bills I guess! Because communications is a trade skill you can use within any industry, and when I moved to Boston, financial services was what was hiring, and by the time I realized I wanted to get out of this soul-sucking quagmire-of-crap industry, I found myself pigeon-holed and nobody else would hire me."

But with great difficulty, and a healthy dose of self-preservation, I manage to bite that back, and he continues. "It seems that for you all to work here, and you're all smart people"—little did he know this is disproved on a daily basis—"it must be special *somehow*."

"Come on, guys, there *is* something special about working here. I mean, I really love it." This comes from Tammy, a less-attractive version of a Stepford wife, married to her small Midwest office. Her voice sounds tinny and forced. An aspiring midlevel manager at one of our regional branch offices that focuses on personal wealth management, she sports huge, permed hair. This, in addition to her hard-won reputation as a slave-driving woman hater who sends emails at three in the morning just to demonstrate she's still working, has earned her the nickname "Medusa" (behind her back, of course—this is financial services, after all). Aside from her hair, nobody takes Medusa very seriously because personal wealth management represents only 20 percent of Investorcap's primarily institutional business model. The thinking behind the strategy was that no matter how rich an individual person was, they were never going to have as much as a really big institution. Thus, personal wealth management and the people who run it are virtually nonexistent on the Investorcap scale of importance.

"I don't know what the future will hold, but whatever it is, I sure hope I'm working here," she continues, and I wonder what limits, if any, this brown-noser has.

I want to snap, "Shut your piehole, Medusa! We're having a moment of truth here…here in the institutional money big leagues." But instead, I glance around nervously: Is there a two-way mirror with our senior management team on the other side? Do I need to start singing the company song? Pledging allegiance to Investor-cap?

Medusa's toe-the-line tone might as well have been a five-alarm warning bell. Honesty ends; rationalized cover-up begins. But even with the specter of Big Brother (real or imagined) hanging over us, after several more hours of brainstorming all we—a roomful of marketing professionals who spend our careers spinning shit into ice cream—can come up with is that surely, there must be *something* special about working here. And frankly, if my honesty had been allowed to keep spewing, I'd happily announce there *isn't*. But my colleagues, obviously less disillusioned and more indoctrinated than I, begin to echo, "Yeah! It *is* special here!" with nothing less than inordinate relief heavy in their voices because it's far more comfortable to join in and keep their jobs without questioning, than to stand apart, question, and eventually be forced to sit with the discomfort of knowing you're a sellout.

Having gotten absolutely nowhere, we're all—well, perhaps except for Medusa—relieved when the meeting ends. We put our faith in the ad agency to come up with a brilliant job campaign. This will entail revving people up while saying absolutely nothing of substance. After all, that's their job.

That night, chefs from the hotel cook us a private dinner at Anderson's Cabin, a one-room log cabin the Ritz made into a chic little chateau so their guests can experience "roughing it." I wonder what John Anderson, the original builder of this then-shack, now-chateau, and one of the seven original bachelors who settled the Gulch in the early 1900s, would think if he could see us, sitting here paying $100 per plate (with an $800 group minimum not including wine, beverages, or the 21% gratuity) so that we can grill our own food, and then go outside to roast s'mores while the staff hands us cookies, chocolate, and marshmallows on fancy Ritz china. Roughing it indeed.

John Anderson would probably roll over in his grave and shit himself laughing, that's what.

In the morning, I check out and glance at the bill that Investorcap prepaid. My room was $980 per night. Which begs the question, what's the difference between this room and the so-called "upgraded" rooms? What were they going to do, plate my toilet seat in gold? Carry me on their backs after they strapped my shoes on my feet? Chew my food for me and then insert it into my gullet like a mama bird does for her chicks? Honestly, what greater luxury could guests need? Did we even really need this level?

Luxurious or not, what business travel teaches me is that it doesn't matter how nice the hotel or what the location, eventually, it's just another place that isn't home.

The grand irony is that when I finally land back in Boston late Friday night, free at last from the gilded cage of corporate travel, the first thing I want to do is go out.

I briefly consider hunkering down on the couch in sweats and no bra, doing absolutely nothing. The even-more fleeting thought that I should ground myself with a little yoga passes even more quickly. Of course I *should* do yoga, maybe even step it up a notch with some breathwork, but I can't. I feel rambunctious. Trapped. Irritated. Frantic. I pace the tiny apartment. I'm hungry, but there's only moldy, months-old food in the fridge. I'm tired, but I'm too wound up to sleep. I'm jet-lagged from being on Denver time and from late, wine-logged nights. Nunnally's jet-lagged on London time and even later nights in front of his laptop. We're both grumpy. It's far from the movie scene I'd envisioned where we're reunited after the unfathomable eternity of a week apart and the sappy music comes on right before the credits roll.

After bickering over whether to order in or go out, we finally end up going out to eat. I literally can't stay in the house.

As we sit at the bar of my favorite Thai-Vietnamese place, I order drink after drink and Nunnally stares at me in a mixture of wonder and horror that I can hold this much alcohol. But my tolerance has increased in the past week out of necessity, because as we all know, I'm a woman in financial services, and the two things that annoy the male execs even more than a female's mere presence are her proclivity to tears and her inability to drink. So I drank. And I drank. And I gluttonously feasted on steak. And I attended meetings and ran meetings and contributed to meetings and participated in "team building" snowmobiling, and I spun faster and faster like a top on amphetamines, thinking only of how much *I just wanted to go home.*

And now I'm home, but having trouble decelerating from 60 to zero in the space of the flight (for once, mercifully not delayed). So I insist we go out to try to create the kind of wing-drag needed to slow me down to a survivable speed as I reenter the atmosphere of my nonwork life.

Of course, by the time I'm sufficiently grounded, it's Monday morning and time to go back to work.

I'm in the usual frantic pursuit of trying to catch up when Betsy sticks her head in my office. "Vicky's on the bathroom floor. The paramedics are on their way. Thought you should know."

I experience a brief post-traumatic flashback to the Great Upchuck Incident.

Minutes later she's taken out on a stretcher. "Just a touch of the flu," Charles says tightly as he walks past. "I've given her the week off."

For the rest of the week, Vicky calls the office a few times a day to chat. "I feel fine!" she coos happily into the phone. "I don't know why Charles is making such a fuss!"

"Yeah, right." Betsy sniffs. "That woman would hurl herself face first into traffic if it'd get her five minutes of attention."

As I'm weaving in and out of traffic and cursing other drivers for not moving faster, Hazel casually mentions that Kim dropped out of the training. *Kim quit?* It's

190

an unexpected development. I focus on driving—*must not rear-end the car in front.*
Given Hazel's revelation about talking with Kim, I arrange my face to try to hide my
overwhelming relief at the news. Thank Krishna! At least one source of crazy has
been eliminated. This momentary reprieve is destroyed as someone cuts me off. I
slam the horn frantically. "What the hell? *Move,* you stupid jerk!"

We arrive moments before the workshop begins, just before the usual hush
sweeps the room signaling Thea's arrival. "Good news, guys! It looks like my karmic debt has finally been settled! No mistakes in this month's workbooks!"

A wave of giggles—*Isn't Thea's battle with the copy place charming?*—and
clapping—*My, how gracious Thea is in her dance with* karma!—greets this news.
*Oh, karma, you adorable rapscallion! Oh Thea, enviable beacon of leadership! If
only we all handled our karma so graciously.*

"Let's open with a chant for *ahimsa,* nonharming of self and others, *satya,*
compassionate truth, and honoring the organic pace of other students' training. We
shouldn't feel tied to the yearlong schedule," Thea says.

I interpret that to mean, don't ask where Kim is. Jaznae's also missing tonight.
Here's hoping she's honoring her "organic pace" as well—and that this pace will call
her away from the program permanently. Or at least until I've graduated.

As we begin, Thea reiterates, for perhaps the hundredth time, the power of the
mind-body connection. "The body is a physical manifestation of the intangibles of
thought and memory."

The insomnia session is especially interesting in its personal applicability. In a
rush of newly found braveness, I ask Thea if I can come in as a client. She looks surprised, but agrees. I'm nervous to do so, but excited to experience what therapeutic
yoga can do.

I leave the room and come back in with the other real clients. We sit on yoga
mats in a neat row opposite Thea and the panel of teacher trainees behind her. I feel
bizarrely disconnected from my class, as I sit here facing them. After attending to the
waves of clients who'd come in for spinal issues and free community classes over
the past several months, I'm now on the receiving end. It's weird that I'm not

perched safely behind Thea, ensconced in the embankment of my fellow trainees. I'm not scribbling intake notes. I feel naked and fidgety without that familiarity. I nervously reband my ponytail and cuff then uncuff my sweatshirt to make up for it.

As is her process, Thea does an intake with each person. Some of these stretch on for quite a while as the clients share details of years of frustration, trials and errors with prescriptions, and home remedies.

I, however, know that later in the debrief, Thea will probably say that these clients are creating—or at least reinforcing—the negative pattern of their insomnia through the telling and retelling of these "stories." It will fall under her theory about needing to create new neurological patterns to combat the "that's just how I am" story they're crafting.

So I'm careful to give just the facts: "I have insomnia." As I make this pronouncement, I try to look yogic and righteous…like I've been working diligently on my individual project to heal the underlying anxiety every single day. Of course, it has actually been banished to the distant reaches of my mind, displaced by my all-consuming job.

As treatment, Thea leads a restorative class. To my unending relief, Hazel and Jessica volunteer to serve as my two assistants. At first, I'm embarrassed that the rest of the class is watching and that Hazel and Jessica's have to wait on me hand and foot. I have the female compulsion to leap up and start pitching in. *Here—let me help you lift those bolsters. Blankets? I'll fold blankets. Oh—this is wrong? Let me move it for you. No problem. I like to help! Really!*

But for once, I consciously try to let go of that. This is their role tonight. It will be my role soon enough. I placate my need to give back by telling myself that maybe I can even repay them by doing a session on them tomorrow. And eventually, I'm able to let go—just a little—and relax into the practice. The quiet confidence of Thea's voice leads us down a path of surrender toward inner stillness.

A sort of deep quietness settles into my body, reverberating through my central nervous system and maybe even up into my brain—my restless, chatty, anxious brain. It's the kind of all-encompassing stillness that breeds soul-deep tranquility for the first time all day, all week. Maybe ever.

As we steep in stillness, Thea intones, "Remember that you always possess the capacity for deeply restful sleep. You were born with this knowledge."

I allow myself to consider that possibility for the first time in my life. The usually endless drive home instead feels effortless—I'm utterly relaxed, body slack, eyes heavy. I crawl into bed, sliding immediately down the slope to unconsciousness. On some level, my body *does* know how to sleep. Maybe I don't have to fight it anymore. Maybe I never did.

Unfortunately, Jaznae is back the next day. My hopes for her organic time off are dashed. She raises her hand as soon as everyone is settled.

"I'm sure you all noticed I was absent last night." Her tone indicates that if you didn't, you should have. What I notice *is* conspicuously absent this morning is her island accent. In its place is a Boston accent. Now that is what I call downright fascinating. "I was participating in a ritual where I manifest art in a graveyard through midnight." She pauses dramatically to let that sink in.

She clearly wants to be asked about it. I would sooner pull my toenails out with pliers. After the group project voted me out, they're all dead to me. In true Italian-old-lady style, I plan to forgive them…never.

Jaznae continues. "So, would it be possible to borrow someone's notes?"

I wonder if she left her fake accent in the graveyard, as I feign busily writing in my notebook. Brinley predictably volunteers her notes to Jaznae, thus demonstrating her community-mindedness to Thea. "And let me know if you have any questions you want to discuss over tea."

"I will consider it." Jaznae says regally, as though she's doing Brinley the favor.

Brinley nods smugly. In her mind, she has clearly won.

I have the fleeting fantasy of walloping both of them with bolsters.

From behind her tea, Thea watches over the flock of us, nodding approvingly. I can tell she's thinking, *Finally, we're a community!* And yet, in spite of her serene smile and tacit approval, she remains completely unapproachable, boundaries up.

I glance at the workshop schedule: over the course of the weekend, there will be ten sessions for various conditions. If it's anything like last month, we'll see another 60 to 100 clients. As Thea initiates intake for each person, I take careful notes and try to anticipate her sequence and language. However, after four hours of hyperfocusing—hearing each person's detailed history and then tending to them, executing all the physical assists, and being ever-watchful—I start to feel overwhelmed...and then totally drained.

According to the schedule, we're supposed to have an hour-long lunch break at noon. From the moment I kicked off my shoes and set up camp in the yoga circle, I've been looking forward to that hour. The possessor of a metabolism that's roughly equivalent to a really spastic, really hungry puppy, I'm pretty much always thinking about, looking forward to, or enjoying my next meal. Maybe I'm kind of shallow, but meals are important to me. So are breaks. Especially breaks from dealing with throngs of people who need to tell you all about their (very serious) problems and then be attended to and cared for. *As in, really taken care of. As in, lift my leg, put it into position, then fetch me a bolster and make 15 micro-adjustments until I'm in slightly less pain.* It's a necessary part of the healing process and I'm happy to help. Except when I'm so hungry all I can think about is getting something to eat before I gnaw off someone's arm.

At 12:30, Thea concludes her last intake and begins the yoga, which makes it clear we aren't getting our break. This is doubly alarming because I'm equal parts starving and worn out. It's not a code-red situation yet—I have no immediate plans to assault anyone and rifle through their bags for food scraps—but it's getting there fast.

But alas, this is not to be. The session drags on until I'm basically drooling on myself, mentally pacing like a caged beast, frenzied from mental overstimulation and physical overexertion.

I even consider asking Summer if I can peel some shoots off whatever the hell she's carrying around and picking at in between assists. I've heard cruciferous greens go well with raw bicep.

I shoot death stares at Thea, hoping she'll feel my desperation—or at least notice my pointed, frantic glances from her to the clock and back again. I'm hoping those glances will prompt her to suddenly remember, "Oh yes, time to feed the yogis!" But she doesn't. I don't want to disrupt the clients' healing by asking aloud. So I suck it up and try not to pout. Or faint. Or leave.

Finally, a full hour late, in between client sessions, Thea laughs breezily, trills some sort of offhand apology, and gives us five minutes to gobble down lunch before the next group comes in. Brinley announces it'll be most rejuvenating to spend the first two minutes in an inversion to release any "toxic vibes" we picked up from the clients and promptly flips up into a headstand. Summer lies on the floor, arms and legs akimbo and sighs heavily, closing her eyes. Gloria and Noemi take legs-up-the-wall pose.

I make an unabashed show of sulking as I scarf down my sandwich, resentful that Thea didn't hold the "boundary" of our lunch hour more strongly by being more disciplined…or utilizing breathwork and *bandhas* to stay grounded, or whatever the yoga phrasing might be. I don't have time to fixate on it, however, because the next set of clients is already coming in. The blend of hyper-focus and physical exertion begins again.

The rest of the weekend passes in a similar blur. There's an endless rotation of clients coming in for sessions for the first six hours, and then we head in to assist the community class. At the door, Thea stops short and holds up one finger. There's a multi-yogi pileup behind her as Brinley, Jaznae, and the rest of the most-ardent admirers who were approximately three inches behind Thea collide.

"Today, we'll all take turns teaching a pose for the first time," she announces. "Won't this be great? Let's allow spontaneity to free the inner teacher within each of us."

I stare. *Is she insane? Did she duck out for a bong hit in her car? What's in that special tea she's always drinking anyway?* Even the thought of teaching without preparation sends me into a fit of anxiety.

"Is there any way I can wait until next month?" I ask, as panic surges.

She considers this for half a second, then smiles her wide, guileless smile. "Okay! But then, you know, you'll have to worry about it for an entire month...."

I size up this elfin yoga master. *Who is she? Innocent guru or calculating manipulator?* It doesn't matter, her point's taken. Best to just get it over with. "I'll teach a sun salutation."

If my voice is peevish, she doesn't acknowledge it. "Good! Good!" She smiles and nods, genuinely happy.

Thea leads the 30-minute drop-in portion of the class as well as the first few poses. "And now Sara will lead you..." she enunciates in her unique, calming way.

I walk to the front, certain that everyone can see my shaking legs. I take a deep breath, face red, and somehow begin—one word after another, one step after another. To my shock, the students are doing as I say and getting where they need to go. The assistants are refining their poses. For all of two minutes, I'm actually leading this class. I'm shocked. Thrilled! I'm doing it! I have the crazy urge to continue teaching instead of passing it back to Thea.

It's amazing how great you can feel about teaching one little pose to a free community class. It's hard to believe how much that can mean. Somehow other accomplishments—putting myself through college, graduating *summa cum laude*, building and running PR programs, climbing the corporate ladder—don't mean as much (at least in this moment) as having taught for the first time.

"And now, I'll turn you over to Thea," I say, smiling goofily.

"Nicely done," Thea says, as I walk past her.

In a state of shock and undiluted joy—both at the accomplishment and the tidbit of praise—I'm practically floating.

Jessica gives me a thumbs-up as she heads to the front. She's up next. For good luck, I do the same, then head into the throng of student bodies.

Unsurprisingly, Jessica's segment is professional and well executed. As I perform an adjustment, I feel inordinately proud of us both.

Thea pops up at my elbow. "See that woman in the purple top?" she murmurs in my ear. "See how she's depressed? How she carries her sadness? Can you see how she's insulating herself from more pain?"

I squint at the utterly average woman in purple, trying to see, but I don't. "Uh...."

Thea steps back and looks at me as though she sees into me too. She waits a long beat. I start sweating. "Hold her feet when she's in *savasana*. There are energy points on the soles."

Honored to be chosen, I nod as though I know what that means and head back into the pack of students.

Happily, with class attendance tripled and trainee enrollment down, there are plenty of students for all of us to assist. There's no racing to make an adjustment, no elbowing, no edging others out. Or maybe most of the elbowers are following their own "organic" pace and not at the training.

Thea brings the class into *savasana*. I meet her gaze and go to the woman in purple. I hold her feet. Thea joins me, kneeling. "Like this," she says gently, cradling the student's right foot in her hands.

I nod and try to imitate what she's doing on the left. The student doesn't move. I wonder how long we'll do this and if it's working. After a few minutes, Thea catches my eye with a small nod and we move away.

After the students have OM-ed and drifted out full of yoga peace, we sit in reflection. I think of the woman in purple and how Thea could see so much and tend to her so kindly. I consider the many clients I saw over the weekend with their myriad conditions. I try to digest how much work we'd done and progress I'd witnessed, and how yoga, which I had entered the training thinking of as a "workout," can, on deep physical, mental, and emotional levels, help and heal people. What I had seen was more profound than muscles merely stretching and strengthening.

But the greatest evolution had taken place within the introduction of each student to the possibility of his or her own inherent and limitless potential. When the mind had quieted enough, students had been able to turn away from hyperactivity or doubt in order to be able to receive those possibilities.

This was a process I understood through my own experience. Similar to how my struggles with insomnia had resulted in self-doubt on some very deep level, and a divorce between what I wanted and what I could make happen, the clients in their own varied ways had also experienced doubts and disassociation. In the same way that quieting my mind and being tended to within my practice had worked to reestablish my faith in my own innate abilities, in the same way that I grew stronger and more capable, I had seen the clients harvest similar benefits.

The question therefore became: Are we each willing to continue this work on our own? Are we willing to take the spark and patiently, devotedly, conscientiously fan the possibility into a daily, lifelong practice?

I renew my commitment to my individual project. I want to work at this. I want to change. I want to move toward a better version of myself.

I think about all that I'm learning and the new ways in which I'm starting to think. Even if I disagree with some of it, I want to share it all with Nunnally. During the lecture portion of workshops, I find myself doodling asterisks next to especially interesting things so that I remember to discuss them with him later that evening. Invariably, however, my brain is so overly full by the time I get home that I'm unable to distill them down into interesting tidbits. I'm simultaneously so overstimulated and physically exhausted that I can't bear the thought of opening up the topics for further discussion. The only thing that seems manageable is silence and wine. Which leaves me one muumuu and a half-smoked cigarette away from an intervention by well-meaning friends and family.

My brain is working furiously just to process this amount of information. Trying to pass it on? Beyond me.

But the fallout is that I feel like I'm leaving Nunnally behind. I've boarded the train for a life-changing journey, and I don't want to leave him standing on the platform. I'm worried that the newly created space between us will yawn into a chasm the size of the Grand Canyon. And how can we maintain our nascent marriage across a chasm? A Grand Canyon-sized chasm? Before my worrying can spiral up, I suggest he attend one of Thea's yoga classes outside the training with me so that he can experience Tri Dosha Yoga for himself.

Unfortunately, the only class near us is an advanced-level class. I decide to keep this information to myself. And if the whole truth must be told, I may secretly be looking forward to watching him struggle a bit. I've been practicing yoga for seven years, devotedly cultivating strength and flexibility, breath and awareness.

He, a devoted, lifelong athlete who was the captain of his college track team and an all-regional middle-distance runner, has, since then, maintained a healthy, if somewhat zealous, devotion to physical fitness. He still works out religiously, burning off work stress with a level of cardiovascular fitness that few other nonprofessionals could manage. So while he can't quite run like he could in the days of his youth, he can tootle out for a ten-mile run and still manage to walk upright the next day, which is more than I could ever manage.

Yoga, however, requires a different sort of endurance, strength, and awareness. You can be an athlete of any kind, but parked in a warrior two combination for a few minutes will get even the strongest thighs trembling. My legs were used to yoga. I'm looking forward to showing Nunnally a thing or two.

I'm proud to introduce him to Thea and feel a rush of excitement as the class begins. I can't wait to glide through the sequence next to my beloved, offering sympathetic smiles and whispered words of encouragement as he labors heavily next to me. I figure it'll be something like watching a fish flop helplessly on dry land. But, you know, a fish that you really love and you know will be back in the water before any real harm's done.

I'm so excited to share my new world with him that I can barely concentrate through the beginning drop-in. "Focus," I command my errant mind. "Be yogic. Don't think about any other students." Stubbornly, my mind continues dancing over to the student on the neighboring mat.

As the class progresses, however, I notice Nunnally is annoyingly good. And as my own struggles ensue (this *is* an advanced class, after all) I battle a mixture of envy, resentment, and pride as Nunnally sails through the class with relative ease.

My arms still strain a bit—even after all these years—under my own weight as I transition from high to low plank. Nunnally, however, eases down gracefully, with, dare I say, damn-near-perfect alignment. We hold low for several deep, slow, *ujjiy* breaths, and as my own breath becomes more intense and labored, the veins in my neck straining a bit, I glance over to find Nunnally looking at me quizzically as he hangs low with seemingly no effort at all—and then even manages an arrow-straight return to high plank, while my alignment suffers, my torso folding slightly, as I still lack the upper body strength for proper execution of such a maneuver.

Of course, I'm proud of him but find myself gritting my teeth. I'd wanted to bring him here so he could get a glimpse of Tri Dosha Yoga, so that he could experience the challenge. And yes...a very small part of me wanted him to be in awe of what I could do that he could not. Instead, he is surprisingly good. Like really, really good! Even more frustrating is that my new self-awareness makes me examine what's driving my desire for him to struggle while also be impressed by me. *It was ego. Darn ego. The anti-yoga.*

Chapter Eighteen

Captain Theatrical Takes Her Show on the Road

Cardio and Other Addictions

O n Friday, Vicky breezes into my office and announces, "Big news: I've decid-ed to leave the company. Nobody's making me go. I'm not being fired or any-thing…no, this is definitely my idea, my choice." The more she insists that she's leaving of her own volition, the more awkward it becomes.

"Yup, I just decided it's time for act two…get it, *act two*? Because I'm in the theater?" Her face crinkles as she cracks herself up. "It's a *theater joke*." She sobers and looks at me resentfully before she continues. "I'm making room in my life for more theater, painting, and men. And my book. And the bonsais of course." She stretches her arms overhead. "*Ahhh*. It just feels so *right*." Smiling, nodding. "Well, the right time is after my stock options and pension plan vest in a few weeks, but don't count on me for any help until then."

A reel of her greatest hits zooms through my brain: takeover-plot hallucina-tions, sequin-costume pictures around the office, fabricated complaints to HR, the Great Upchuck Incident, the poem in San Diego, her bad-smell confessions….

"Well Vicky, I wish you the best," I manage to say—barely.

"You don't seem shocked," she notes, slumping. Clearly she wanted a dramatic response to her big news.

"I'm just taking it all in," I say instead as an overwhelming sense of relief courses through my body. I knew it would eventually be her or me who had to go. I've emerged victorious. DiVello: one, Captain Theatrical: zip.

Betsy walks by the glass wall of my office and mimes the Snoopy happy dance behind Vicky. It culminates in a ta-tas-shaking finale directly above Vicky's head. I bite my bottom lip hard to keep from laughing. Good thing Vicky can't see this—as a final act of authority she'd probably report Betsy for inappropriate possession of mammaries.

Vicky breezes out to continue spreading news of her impending departure. From the expectant look on her face, I can tell she hopes for more-validating, "Oh gosh, *no!*" responses. I gleefully kick off my heels and recount the whole thing to Nunnally in an excited whisper over the phone, allowing myself a buoying surge of optimism that it's who I've worked for and not what I do that's been making me so unhappy. The prospect of a new (and hopefully sane) boss is an unexpected but welcome boon.

"This weekend, we are continuing our studies on yoga's healing effects on the emotional body," Thea says.

I try to mentally change gears, leaving the office and gleeful thoughts of Vicky's departure behind. I also try to steer clear of thoughts about how I was here only 20 days ago. Seeing endless rounds of clients. Without any breaks. And no time off for lunch. Not that I'm bitter. Or petty. Or overly obsessed with lunch breaks, of course.

Thea continues. "Remember—it's the yoga and the students themselves who create their own healing. You guys don't need a background in psychotherapy. If a client wants to say something to a yoga therapist, it's heard, but not 'worked through.'"

Immediately, I wonder what sort of "healing" we're getting into now? In spite of her assurance, I don't know what to do in a needs-healing situation—smile? nod? *OM?* What does it mean to "hear but not work through" something?

"The first thing we'll do is map our *samskarras,*" Thea says. "*Samskarras* are the patterns in our lives—within ourselves and everyone we interact with. We'll start by sketching our triggers and the resulting patterns in our notebooks."

After a thorough two-to-three-second consideration, I decide to focus on work stress. It highjacks you, clobbers you over the head, and drags you down into dark, murky water as you gasp for air and futilely try to resist. It leaves you wide awake, your brain churning, your eyes staring at the ceiling fan at four in the morning whereas other stress can usually be assuaged with a glass of wine. Or five.

Thea instructs us to pair off and I look around for Jessica but find that she's already hunched over a notebook, apparently partnering with a drop-in student who's not part of the training. During the requisite introductions she'd announced to the class that she was feeling anxious because she'd driven here on just half a tank of gas, and, fearful of running out, had put her car into neutral and coasted down all the hills. It was then that I'd made a mental note to steer clear. If we weren't aligned on the basic importance of getting gas on a road trip, where could we go from there?

Hazel, too, is already taken. Both my regular partners are already partnered off? Is anyone besides Jaznae or Brinley not taken? As though psychic, I see the two of them pair off at that moment. I scan the room, looking for *anyone*.

"Wanna be partners?"

I turn toward the voice and find myself face-to-face with Harper, the grad student from Tennessee. "Sure," I say.

She volunteers to go first. "My *samskarra* is that I'm addicted to people, pills, smoking, and booze," she announces and then just stares at me.

I stare back, wondering again if I agree with Thea's theory that you don't need a psychotherapy background for this. What am I supposed to do—suggest child's pose?

"It starts with a craving for one of these things," she clarifies, pointing to her notebook. "So at night I'm alone. I'm bored. So I start craving a guy…or a girl," she glances at me to make sure I've gotten the bisexual reference.

I nod to show that I have.

She continues. "Or getting high…like really bad. Even if I know it isn't good for me. So then I think, 'I shouldn't call him. And I shouldn't smoke. It makes me depressed and lethargic.' So then I try not to. But then I have a drink, which turns into ten. But then the drinks aren't enough so I take pills or I smoke. And then I feel like, 'Well, shit, why shouldn't I have what I want? To hell with it.' So then I drink more, and then I call someone really bad for me and then I do something really irresponsible. And then I feel really, really, REALLY bad about myself the next day. Like, 'What was I thinking? I'm such a loser.' And I get really down on myself. So then I drink or take more pills or smoke or whatever to feel better." She shrugs. "It's a cycle."

I look at my notes, hoping they will reveal some magical insight, hoping that something beyond what I scribbled will appear, telling me how to help her. Of course, no such thing is there, and I flash back to the refrain I've reverted to so often throughout this training: *I'm here for the yoga. Yoga anyone? Yoga?*

"Hmm…well, where do you think you might be able to make an intervention?" I ask, as per Thea's instructions. My voice sounds formal, stupidly clinical, even to my own ears. I clear my throat nervously. I wish I sounded more natural, but I feel completely, utterly, even *woefully* unprepared.

She shrugs again. "I dunno. That's why I mapped it out." She looks at me, completely open, not embarrassed, waiting for me to help her.

I study her diagram. I don't see one either—aside from the obvious idea of not allowing one beer to turn into ten, which seems to be the gateway that leads to pill-popping and dangerous sexual behavior. Isn't that the hallmark of addiction, though? Not being able to stop at just one? Suggesting the obvious—that she only have one drink (or not drink at all)—is basically like telling anyone with an addiction, "Well…just…*stop already*." If it was that easy, people wouldn't have addictions, right? Feeling desperate, I suggest we go ask Thea. Harper agreeably tags along behind me as I plow toward the other side of the room.

Of course, Brinley, blatantly disregarding Thea's boundaries, is already talking to her. I think I can guess the topic. The usual crowd of admirers sits in a semicircle around them, avidly taking notes. I want to administer a round of swift kicks to them all.

Thanks to Brinley and the rest of the devotees, we don't make it up to Thea in time before she restarts her lecture. I'm worried about Harper. "You should definitely ask Thea later," I say.

She shrugs noncommittally. "Sorry we didn't get to yours," she says.

"It's fine. Mine were stupid, really. I just mapped out stress with work." That sounds inadequate compared to Harper's. I hurry to add something—anything—else. "I also get irritated with my husband because he's always late—like when he says he'll meet me at a certain time and then I end up waiting for hours, while he's stuck at work or something. So it's annoying, but that's all." Damn. Mine still sound silly.

"You sure have a lot of expectations about your job and partner," Harper says, offhandedly, gently correcting my non-yogic, gender-specific spousal reference.

I pause, mildly offended. Then I wonder: *Is she right?* Maybe I do—and if I'd just let go of expecting work to be less stressful or Nunnally to be on time, I wouldn't be irritated when things didn't work out as I had expected. Maybe Harper has a point.

Then again, if you don't expect someone to be on time, then how would any of us make plans? Like, *I'll see you at Starbucks...whenever?*

Interestingly, research shows that a person's physiological and mental response to stress doesn't vary between "real" stress (death of a loved one, loss of job, etc.) and "self-perceived" stress ("I have too many dinner plans"). If a person perceives their situation as stressful, the body reacts as though the stress is real—experiencing anxiety, depression, insomnia, weight gain, etc. There seems to be a lesson in there somewhere, but I'm too tired to decipher what it is.

Thea resumes lecturing, but I can't stop thinking about Harper. With the enormity of her addiction *samskarra* laid out so plainly at my feet, I wonder if Thea's sphinxlike edict that yoga and students' own work are the keys to healing really are enough to help with something as serious as an addiction. Clearly, Harper already does yoga. She's even doing *yoga teacher training*. And yet she still battles her addictions and self-destructive patterns. So what's Thea's answer to that? More yoga?

Private sessions? I'd like to ask, but won't of course because that would reveal Harper's addictions to the rest of the class. I hope she'll confide in Thea.

After more lecture, Thea dismisses us for the evening and I start to gather my notebook, workshop handouts, and collection of pens—blue and black ink options, and a veritable rainbow of highlighters—and put them in my bag. Delicate bare feet appear in front of me. I look up and Thea's standing over me. "For your *samskarra* work this weekend, why don't you focus on your group project situation and what that stirred up for you," she suggests quietly. Suddenly my work stress and issues with Nunnally's chronic disregard for punctuality recede into dots in my rearview mirror. Just as Thea had discarded my urban yogini idea and put in front of me the work of resolving my anxiety, she once again was swooping in with a reality call. As always, I'm in awe of her astute insights.

This isn't going to be an easy weekend, I think as I drive home. It isn't until I'm lying awake in a frustratingly wide-eyed bout of insomnia that I consider the bizarre incongruity that for a therapist who seems to advocate only the healing properties of yoga, the *samskarra*-mapping partner work, greatest scar-sharing exercise, and homework centered around identifying and analyzing our interpersonal dynamics seemed an awful lot like…therapy.

The next day, Thea announces that we're tackling depression and gives a brief overview of the condition.

Depression, which is technically the hypoarousal (or lowered state of functioning) of the nervous system, leads to lowered levels of norepinephrine and epinephrine—the chemicals associated with happiness. Exercise has been proven to boost these chemicals in the brain, which is why people feel good afterward, or are sometimes said to experience a "runner's high."

"However," Thea cautions sternly, "most bodies aren't built to run long term without injury, and cardio in general is addictive. *Vinyasa* yoga—and especially core work—is still a good workout for the cardiovascular system and boosts the production of the neurochemicals that elevate mood, but *safely*—without overstimulating your system."

I'm taking notes as rapidly as she's speaking but come to a screeching halt at that. *Is Thea suggesting that yoga be our only form of exercise?* What about the fact that the heart is a muscle that, like any muscle, needs to be strengthened through exercise, which research indicates means significantly elevating your heart rate? While yoga is a wonderful addition to my life—providing a deep sense of relaxation, improved flexibility, as well as overall toning and strengthening—I still run and use the elliptical machine for cardiovascular exercise.

Remembering my resolution to speak up when I have something to say, I raise my hand. "What about the standard recommendation for 30 minutes of cardio five days a week? Doesn't exercise play a part in our cardiovascular health?"

Thea leans back slightly and crosses her ankles. *Uh-oh.*

"Cardio is *very* addictive," she repeats. "And because it mimics the stress response—elevated heart and respiration rates—if you tend toward anxiety, I wouldn't recommend it. For instance, I would *never* have you or Jessica anywhere near a treadmill."

Jessica, who's currently training for the Boston Marathon, and I exchange guilty glances. Apparently, we have been singled out as the evil cardio addicts in a room full of tranquil yogis.

For a moment, I feel a bit betrayed. I had raised this question as a student, not as an anxiety-sufferer. Second, I had confided my anxiety to Thea privately in my study questions and in my progress reports on my yearlong project. To be called out publicly, in front of the rest of the trainees who, with their holier-than-OM vibe, don't know that I have anxiety, feels like being outed against my will.

I take a deep breath and try not to mind. *It's okay. Surely, I'm not the only one here to have anxiety,* I tell myself. Then again, considering who I'm dealing with—these chanting, meditating, I-don't-work-a-real-job yogis…and considering that I am literally the only one who has a high-stress corporate job and lives in the city, in my own condo, with my husband instead of in a yurt on a commune...well, maybe I am the only one.

"Trying to burn off anxiety or power through depression with cardio and without yoga will eventually result in adrenal exhaustion. Anxiety already overstimulates the production of cortisol, the stress hormone—and, over time, probably results in injuring most bodies."

"Yeah, you might as well do power yoga," Brinley says with a derisive snort.

Kim rolls her eyes. "Seriously."

I redden. I'd started in power yoga and spent years benefiting richly from it. Yes, I'd since found more depth and richness in slower yoga, but that didn't mean *ashtanga* was to be derided. I think about saying this, but don't have the energy for a second debate.

As usual, there's a rush to support Thea. The rest of the class is nodding fervently, murmuring their agreement robotically, and taking notes in their decorative Indian-themed journals on the perils of non-yogic cardio.

I feel like it's me (and Jessica) against a roomful of people, most importantly our teacher, who holds an advanced degree and knows more about the physical and mental aspects of anxiety and depression than I ever will. Singled out, I get stubborn. I'm not ready to let it go. "Yoga just doesn't seem like enough of a workout," I finally manage, which sounds weak even to my own ears. "I mean, I love it and I couldn't do without it, but in terms of staying fit physically and cardiovascularly...." My voice trails off. "What about the heart? And lungs?"

Thea, as ever, is impenetrable. "Let's put it to the class," she suggests maddeningly.

Here it is again, that most loathsome of teaching tricks: the class vote. Never a fan of this technique, I especially hate it here because it has already been proven that nobody except me will ever, *ever* dare to oppose Thea. My fellow teacher-trainees either just happen to be coincidentally in agreement with every blessed concept Thea has ever uttered, or are a herd of lemmings, and I'm about the only mutant in the room willing to suggest stepping back from the cliff for a moment to pause and consider other options. And just to top it off, like most human beings in a student's subservient position, I find there is nothing more obnoxious than not being addressed directly, but instead being shamed by the larger democracy.

"What does everyone think?" Thea asks.

There is a resounding chorus of, "Oh, absolutely, Thea!" and "Definitely!" and "Please! Your classes are hard enough! I can barely get through!" and "I drink the nectar of wisdom from the overflowing cistern of your psyche!"

Okay, maybe I imagined that last one. But the overwhelmingly obsequious nature of the all-encompassing agreement with Thea stops barely short of that mark.

"So," Thea continues relentlessly, "when I have you on one leg for eight or ten breaths…do you guys feel it?"

Janet is nodding so hard her head threatens to come off. "Oh Lord, yes! My heart is just thundering! Thundering! Pounding in my chest!"

"Yoga is the only safe form of exercise for me," Brinley chimes in, placing a hand on her abdomen. "I'd never even consider cardio." She shoots a patronizing look toward Jessica and me.

"Yoga awakens my inner life force and I allow this awakening to heal and harmonize my art and my life," Jaznae tells the class, deliberately looking into the distance in what can only be described as a pose that begs to be looked at.

"I feel the same way about my freecycle art," Gloria adds enthusiastically. She's so eager to join in with the group that I feel bad when everyone ignores her.

Summer, who went running with Jessica and me during the immersion, smiles sweetly and says nothing. Hazel also stays silent. Everyone else continues in a mad race to agree with Thea.

"Well, obviously, some poses are really challenging and I feel it too…for a few breaths," I hasten to add, wanting to end the disagreement. "But in terms of it being comparable to the recommended amount of weekly exercise? No, yoga's not even close. Which is why I supplement with some cardio a few days a week. I feel like it's good for the whole cardiovascular system. And it relieves my stress."

Jessica, cherished fellow cardio criminal, jumps in. "Absolutely. When I'm really stressed, running helps." Stony silence greets this. "Plus it just feels good, and it's good for me," Jessica adds.

Thea levels us with her gaze. "Again, I wouldn't recommend running for *either* of you. Not with your levels of anxiety. I'll say it again: running, which elevates your heart rate, leaves you out of breath, and sends cortisol coursing through your system, can be mistaken by the body as anxiety and can eventually lead to adrenal exhaustion. Next time, try sitting with your discomfort and see what comes up instead of trying to run away from...whatever you're running away from." She looks away and the discussion is ended.

Defiantly, I want to run out of the room and take a flying leap onto the nearest treadmill just because I can, but at the same time I feel the need to hide my cardio "addiction" from Thea and the yogis. Or, as I now think of them, the bogis—bogus yogis. I resent that Thea unfairly twisted my moderate, healthy cardio routine into "running away from my problems." It's a gross distortion of the truth. But once again, she has pointedly cut off the discourse.

Apparently that's all there will be on this subject. I'm impotent and unable to defend myself.

Chapter Nineteen
Emails Gone Wild

Irrefutable Proof of Reincarnation:
The #@!% Group Projects Rise Again

There's a group of sales guys in The Meat's office, and the energetic current of juicy gossip is zinging around the floor. Betsy, who always has the scoop, informs me that one of the sales guys had accidentally emailed the company's entire client list with an extraordinarily detailed sexual fantasy. Allegedly, it involved a horse. Charles had promptly called the equine fan into his office and docked his bonus—said to be over $500,000. He would, however, remain employed. Sales guys could pretty much get away with anything.

The Meat's unapologetically loud voice booms down the hall. "*Dude*! A freaking *horse*!"

Raucous laughter erupts just as my phone rings. "This is Sara," I say, rolling my eyes and turning away from my view of The Meat's office.

"Hey!" Hanna says. "What're you up to?"

I glance back at the guys across the way, still hanging out. "The usual. Working. Trying to get everything done before five."

"I won't keep you then. I'm just calling to see if you want to have dinner with Annie and me tonight."

My heart sinks. "I can't. I have training." I realize I haven't kept my resolution to see my sisters. I haven't seen them since Christmas. "How about Sunday night after the workshop ends?"

"No, you'll be too tired."

Unfortunately, that's probably true. "Monday?"

"No, I have class," Hanna says, already working on her master's. "You seem really stressed anyway. Let's just take a rain check."

"Are you sure that's okay?" I ask, secretly relieved, but feeling guilty.

"Sure," Hanna says, but it's clear she doesn't mean it.

Thea leads the chant and I find myself looking forward to it, raising my voice more confidently. Somehow chanting isn't as scary as it used to be. I even dare to think I harmonize fairly well with the group.

The familiarity of the ritual, as well as the rhythms of each particular chant, of the now-recognizable Sanskrit words, is comforting. Closing my eyes and chanting for *ahimsa,* kindness, used to seem pretty weird. Now it's become almost as familiar as the taste of Nana's chicken soup or the Dial soap smell of her bathroom.

"Let's examine the concept of striving within our practices," Thea says. "If you try to yank your body into something, it rebels. If you coax it slowly and patiently, it thanks you, and releases. Let's take a minute to reflect on which approach we default to."

I avoid her gaze, which, once again, seems to be lingering accusingly on me. Her uncanny ability to home in on issues is unnerving. She's like a heat-seeking missile and my overdoing, overstriving, overly high expectations are in her crosshairs. Melting under the intensity of her gaze, I try to dig up these issues. Why *do* I demand that my hamstrings lengthen, my hips open to full lotus, my inversions tip up seamlessly? It's so much more yogic to slowly, patiently persuade.

Why? *Why?* Because I'm an anxious, impatient perfectionist. *Duh.*

Ah yes, my faithful ol' sidekicks. But identifying these problems isn't enough. Even I can see there's a better way to be. There's a better way to be in my practice, and no doubt off the mat as well, extending to job, Nunnally, family, and friends. What are my expectations and what anxiety do I create around them? How would my *experience* of events be different if I altered my approach?

I'm challenging how I think and what I do, and I like that. The importance of this is not lost on me.

"Before we get to the syllabus, I want to remind everyone to keep working on their knowledge of Sanskrit. You should know every pose by its native name," Thea says.

My anxiety spikes. I don't have the Sanskrit names memorized.

"Now," Thea says, "let's spend some time on how we work with students with various levels of experience. Then we'll move on to how to teach ourselves within our home practices."

I feel guilty at the mention of a home practice. I've never had one. My last apartment was a 300-square-foot walk-up. I could stand in the living area and nearly touch the side walls with my fingertips. My current condo, at 600 square feet (double the size of my previous single-gal abode—a palace! practically an estate! a small town!), shrank magically when Nunnally moved in. And even back when it seemed relatively palatial, there certainly was no yoga studio. There wasn't even a dining room.

True, there was room for a yoga mat. There's always room for a mat. But I hadn't cultivated a home practice because the few times I tried had been…well, boring and lonely. Solitude is the innate, necessary nature of a home practice. But I hadn't realized that that meant it would feel lonely. And to feel lonely is un-fun. And un-fun is the ender of new endeavors.

It's that same desire for camaraderie and the boundaries of being in a quasi-work environment that drives laptop users to coffee shops. You know those people probably *could* be working at home, and maybe they'd even work better in solitude and silence, but they *choose* not to.

Of course, that's assuming their homes are empty and silent. For all I know, they could be escaping 32 roommates, newborn quintuplets, or a barnyard cacophony of various other chaotic events. But in a far more likely scenario, cafe-goers go to cafes for the same reasons yoga practitioners go to classes: because there's a certain energy and companionship there. In classes, there's also the structure and support of a teacher guiding you. Sure, you can ignore the teacher. You can always ignore the teacher. But it's easier to let the teacher guide you than it is to think up your own practice and discipline yourself to stick to it.

I pull my brain back to the present as Thea transitions to the pace of our practices as a tool for re-patterning. "Just as we work on alignment within poses, we must be mindful to attune to our inner alignment as well. And to do the work to evolve beyond 'how we are.' For instance, anxious students will gravitate toward faster practices."

She pauses and I could be paranoid, but I could swear her gaze lingers on me before it skips over to Jessica.

"But utilizing tools like sequencing and adjusting speed can provide us the chance to become different versions of ourselves...more-balanced versions," Thea finishes.

I'll admit (to myself) that it does feel good and right and very, very normal when I go fast: think fast, drive fast, practice fast, work fast. In fact, over the course of my career, I've been continually rewarded and promoted for my ability to work quickly and multitask.

Like most modern-day women, I'm a grade-A multitasking master. A professional at endlessly dividing my attention. A veritable genius at spreading myself too thin! While cooking dinner with all four burners going on the stove, I can still simultaneously maintain an in-depth phone conversation, apply mascara between washing dishes, and all the while, dust with my foot and pantomime instructions to Nunnally who's on his cell giving directions to a lost guest and looking just as lost himself as he watches the whirling dervish of activity that was once his wife.

To consider the idea that, although it feels both normal and right to me, it may, in fact, be neither, gives me serious pause. And just like that, once again, I'm impressed at Thea's provocative questions and insights.

Where would it leave me if I didn't go fast? If I went slowly, focusing on one thing at a time, how would I accomplish everything? How would I hold down my job, travel as much as I do, get to the gym, maintain my marriage, keep up my friendships, preserve my familial relationships, get everything done at home, and still manage to get a few hours of sleep? How do my friends with kids do all that *and* raise the next generation?

The next morning starts with a Mysore practice, which basically means, you do whatever the hell you want. Yogically, of course.

If we were practicing in the *ashtanga* tradition (the power yoga style in which I started), it would be more like a contortionism contest with everyone trying to out-yoga, out-do, and outlast the people next to them. Instead, it's more of an I'm-the-most-yogic competition where everyone is trying to out-Zen each other.

We break for lunch, which was originally scheduled to be 45 minutes, but Thea overshoots the time again and leaves us only ten.

Again, I'm irritated. And not in the *oh, la-di-da, I'm annoyed but I can manage* way. But in the *I'm-so-frigging-starving-I-want-to-kick-your-ass* way. I look around. Surely, I can't be the only one who thinks this condensed break is woefully inadequate. Surely I'm not the only one who can barely inhale her lunch that fast—let alone go anywhere to buy lunch, consume it, and get back here. But the rate of food-consumption is only part of the problem. Ten minutes isn't nearly enough time to aerate my brain sufficiently to compensate for the amount of information we're supposed to absorb. But of course, I know what will happen if I voice these complaints. I can't bear the idea of the bogis buttering up to Thea, swearing up and down that *of course* ten minutes is enough—*oodles and oodles of time! What kind of a loser would possibly need more?*

I decide to discuss it in the evaluation portion of my homework.

"Okay! Group projects! Who wants to go first?" Thea announces.

My heart plummets. Here it is: irrefutable evidence of reincarnation. Will this topic ever just die?

Jessica and Noemi make their way to the front.

"Just the two of you?" Thea asks.

"We used to have Harper, but she dropped out," Jessica says. My heart drops. I hope Harper shared her addictions with Thea. I look at Thea but her face is impassive.

"Our project was a survey of different styles of yoga. We sampled classes and rated everything from use of Sanskrit, to level of physical challenge." Jessica says, passing out bound copies of the results to everyone.

Thea, looking thoroughly unimpressed, nods and says nothing.

Gloria, Hazel, and Summer go next.

"We were going to do a book of poses," Summer begins.

"There was going to be a book!" Gloria echoes, chipper as ever.

"It was going to be great," Summer continues. "Like showing, like, every single pose in all of yoga."

"Every pose!" Gloria chimes in. "A beautiful, real book! And you'd all get copies."

"But somehow…we couldn't get it together." Summer says.

"Just. Could. Not," Gloria says, making the cut-off motion with her hands.

"I started to feel like Hazel and Gloria weren't listening to my ideas because I'm, like, so much younger than they are," Summer says. "And I was like 'um…why aren't you guys, like, listening to my ideas? Is it because I'm, like, so much younger than you are?'"

Hazel, who, as per usual, looks totally calm in the midst of this chaos, finally speaks up, "I felt really bad when I realized I was making Summer feel like that. So I apologized. And then we all talked and decided to ask Thea about it, but Thea said we should work it out among ourselves. So we all talked about it again, and I apologized again for my age discrimination."

"And *that* is our project," Summer concludes.

"*We* are our project," Gloria adds.

"We were going to do a book," Summer says over her.

"A *beautiful* book," Gloria says over Summer.

"But instead we are our project."

"We—" Gloria does a wrist and arm circling dance gesture—"are our project." She bows her head over her hands in prayer. Summer and Hazel follow suit.

216

"Isn't that *so cool*!" Thea exclaims, sounding more impressed and excited than I've ever known her to sound. "Wow. They really got in there and dealt with their *samskarras* and look! What a powerful project! What an example of self-evolution! Now *that* is yoga!"

She looks pointedly at my group: Jaznae, Janet, and me. Jaznae looks supremely unconcerned and self-righteous. Janet looks like she might cry. I feel ashamed, as though I've failed somehow. Kim isn't there to react.

Brinley raises her hand. "We'll go next, Thea."

She and Noemi, who is apparently involved in two group projects—which I didn't know was even a possibility—move to the front of the room, and I wonder how much I should bet on the likelihood that this involves wandering organs.

"We're also our project," Brinley says. "Originally, I wanted to do my project on making peace with my wandering spleen...."

And there it is.

"But then I started talking to Noemi." Brinley smiles over at her.

"I was concerned as a long-distance student about how I'd participate in a group project. But then I ended up doing two! This one came about after Brinley and I got talking after a workshop and we decided to partner too," Noemi says.

"Which has been *wonderful*," Brinley picks up, "just *wonderful*. Our project has consisted of emailing thoughts about the training. And we've gotten together for tea."

I wait for more, but it doesn't come. Tea and emailing. *Wow.* By that standard, I've completed group projects with both Jessica and Hazel. *Why, look! I got to be in groups with my friends after all!*

The rest of the presentations continue in this vein. I wonder what will happen when we get to our fractured semblance of a group. But Thea never calls on us.

Chapter Twenty
The Inherent Safety of Corporate Identity

...And the Elusive State of Yoga-ness

Later that week, Nunnally and I head to his friend Brian's birthday party, which is being held in a private room at a bar downtown. I demand we stand outside while I finish an email to Charles. As usual, he's freaking out because he doesn't read his email. He makes Betsy check it and then read it to him...an arrangement that doesn't work so well on weekends. I reassure him via her that everything is in order, and resend the confirmations I'd already sent a week ago. Of course, there is the almost-certain possibility that he won't read this email either, but I'm not calling him on a Saturday night.

As I press each key with unnecessary force, Nunnally mentions that his ex-girlfriend, who I've never met, is also expected to be there. Preoccupied, I hit send, touch up my lip gloss, and head in, barely registering this tidbit of information. Inside, we make the obligatory social rounds. "I'm going to the ladies room and then the bar," I tell Nunnally. "What do you want—vodka and soda?"

"Thanks, sugar mama," Nunnally jokes.

When I get to the bar, it's six deep. "Wow, I don't think I even know this many people," the guy next to me says.

I laugh, thinking our wedding was smaller. "Me neither. So...how do you know Brian?"

"We work together," he says, and I digest the fact that he, like Brian and I, works in finance too. "What about you?"

"My husband went to college with him," I say, leaving out that I also work in the financial industry. I don't want to talk shop. Peripherally, I see movement and turn to face a woman wearing a knee-length skirt and a bad attitude. Standing at a distance that most people would consider far too close, she looks me over from head to toe, then zeroes in to stare straight into my eyes. Well, straight *up* into my eyes. Her head doesn't clear my chin. Next to her, I'm a towering giantess. It's an all-too familiar feeling.

"I'm a lawyer," she spits out. "What are you?"

What am I? I'm taken aback at this onslaught is what I am. Who is this person and what's with the aggressive hostility? My brain kicks into overdrive, and realization dawns as the *Jaws'* music starts: this must be Nunnally's ex-girlfriend. Instinctively, I rise to my full height and puff up my hypothetical feathers. "I'm the head of public relations for Investorcap, a 750-billion-dollar international financial services company." I clarify since she doesn't work in the industry. Suddenly the job I hate provides a sturdy level of defense and a definite level of pride in the face of this assault. I take refuge in both. Fresh off a training weekend, it flashes through my mind that "yoga teacher" just would not have the same panache.

Only later will I kick myself for not saying something cool like, "Um…I'm *human*. What are *you*?" It's an unfortunate trait to only think of suave retorts at three in the morning, well after the time that they would've come in handy.

"Well…where do you *live*?"

"The South End," I say, watching her jealousy ratchet up a notch.

"Well, I'm an attorney," she repeats, "a *tax attorney*."

Since we're back to careering each other, I assume I won the address contest.

"Oh. Does that mean you sit in an office all day reading the tax code? Bummer." And with that, I fail to take my yoga off the mat and find that the slippery snake of pettiness is still alive and well within me.

Her brows knit furiously. "It's not a bummer! It's fabulous!" She is one shrill note away from stomping her penny loafer.

The bud of my non-yogic pettiness blossoms into a full non-lotus, as I note premature wrinkling around her eyes and mouth, probably from unprotected sun exposure—or excessive scowling.

Brian's co-worker speaks up. "I've actually been telling her she should've gone into finance," he says, gesturing to Nunnally's ex, "the money's good without the law school debt or billable hours."

I look from him to her and back again. *Why would this guy...?* I realize that I've been unwittingly chatting with the current boyfriend of Nunnally's ex-girlfriend, her Nunnally 2.0. I follow this train of thought to its logical next step: I was just confronted by myself, version 1.0.

The new boyfriend looks appraisingly at me. "You must be really smart if you're the head of PR at Investorcap. They're major."

I smile demurely and shake my head, modestly denying the compliment, as Nunnally's ex pivots on her heel and stomps off, silenced at last. If she were a cartoon, smoke would be coming out of her ears. For once, I try to play it cool, which is obviously not my natural tendency, but inside I'm enjoying the smackdown, just a little.

Yes, the state of being yogic is elusive indeed.

Later that night as I try to fall asleep, the encounter replays over and over in my mind. Vitriol is always unnerving. I wish I could just let it go and be unaffected, but I can't. I'm sensitive. This stuff bothers me. Clearly, from her brief yet aggressive interrogation, Taxerina places a great deal of value on profession, title, and neighborhood—pretty much the opposite of everything the yoga path values.

And yet, what had I, who was supposedly pursuing the yogic path, done when confronted? Why, I dumpster-dove straight into ego, material possessions, and combative wordplay of course! And beyond that, I'd retreated back to my corporate identity like a coward.

I hated that I had done this, but I had. When I needed it, despite dismissing and degrading it when I didn't, I still had the corporate world to use as armor—to shield me and give me ammunition to volley back at Nunnally's ex-girlfriend. In case of an emergency, I still had corporate weapons with which to duel.

But what if I didn't have that corporate fallback? What if I, like everyone else in my class, was on my way toward becoming a yoga teacher instead of just using this as a tiny meaningful morsel to supplement my meaningless corporate job? What if, like the rest of my class, all I'd had to retort back was, "Um…actually, I'm uh…a yoga teacher"?

Buh-DUM-dum-*splat*.

Yoga is something that, notwithstanding my failure to uphold its virtues in my unfortunate encounter with Taxerina, I believe in. Inside, I'd be proud of this statement. But with no formal educational requirement and what can only be described as dismal prospects for earnings potential, how would that stack up against "I'm a lawyer"?

It wouldn't. It would earn me a victorious, withering look from Taxerina as she sashayed off, certain that my husband had unambiguously traded down. And it would've left me feeling lowered, a loser in that match, a nonentity in the eyes of this woman who was a microcosm of the broader non-yoga world that is…oh wait…the majority of the developed world's population. Nobody hopes that their kid will grow up to teach yoga. But how many mothers have coddled dreams of raising little doctors or lawyers?

I said I dismissed narcissistic materialism, but on some level I bought into it.

I already knew that I harbored the *samskarra* of not staying present within my own practice, failing to allow the edges of my mat to provide veritable walls beyond which I was not supposed to peek. But I now sensed I had an off-the-mat parallel habit of peeking at my friends' lives. And that was no more beneficial than watching my yoga neighbor.

Peer pressure is a concept that, in abstract, we breezily dismiss—*No, Mom, if my friends jump off a bridge of course I won't jump too*—but in its more subtle and subversive iterations, when *everyone* you know works eight to five in big tall buildings and has no time with their spouses or family or friends…when everyone you know leads a fast-paced lifestyle with no time to tune in to their bodies, health, or well-being, when everyone you know wants the big window office and the promotion it entails, then it normalizes the fact that your life looks like that too. You think, "Well, this is how it is for *everyone,*" and somehow you feel better about it.

I know I shouldn't care what anyone else thinks or does. But clearly I still had enough ego that I *did* care what others thought, what Taxerina thought, what the other people listening around us at the party thought. And it had felt good to be able to have a "respectable" comeback—"respectable" as defined by those who buy into valuing corporate life, who place importance on climbing the corporate hierarchy. Maybe I, too, had let myself get swept up into believing that titles and offices with a view and all the other corporate trappings actually meant something. Or maybe I was innately more competitive and less "yogic" than I would've liked, but I was relieved to have a bitchy retort. Hell, I had actually reveled in my comeback.

Despite dismissing it, denying any value in it, even mocking it most of the time, there was also a part of me that was proud of what I'd been able to achieve in this world that I ultimately didn't buy into. I was proud of the level to which I'd climbed on a ladder I criticized as meaningless and corrupt. Despite the intrinsic worthlessness of what I did, I was conversely proud to be able to say to the aggressive Taxerina, "Who *me*? I'm the Director of Public Relations of a 750-Billion-Dollar International Financial Services Company."

And yes, in my delivery, I'd verbally capitalized not only my title, but the whole damn thing. Take that, Taxerina! *Snizzap!*

But that was exactly the problem. Beyond Taxerina's intense competitiveness and confrontational manner, which was certainly off-putting, the real issue was my even-more-concerning response—my need to swell up and duel with her on the battlefield of bitchiness. My response and all it entailed was way worse.

I consider what retort I'd use—*or lack*—if I didn't have my job and title, in the unlikely event that this situation ever presents itself again. But given that it had only happened once in my life so far, the chances of a recurrence are probably slim.

I'm forced to admit that what I'm really worried about is my own view of myself and my place in, and relationship to, the world. And my worry is this: If what you do doesn't matter to the majority of the population and you instead choose to relinquish the trappings of success that that same majority values and follow a path that is not only known by few but tread by fewer still…*but* you don't go live in a hut

in the Himalayas and instead dwell among the majority in a big city as an outsider...
then do you still exist at all?

If you aren't *acknowledged*, are you still there?

I think of what my Aunt Joan would do if she were in my place. She would've
been completely unaffected. She wouldn't have even bothered to recount the interaction. It takes a lot to get under her skin and this wouldn't have even registered. My
aunt is the most yogic person I know, yogis included, and she barely practices yoga
on the mat. And while I've always been aware of how much I've benefited from her
wisdom, thoughtfulness, and compassion, I'd never thought of those traits as specifically *yogic*. Because, until now, I had wrongly thought of yoga as a physical practice.

Unfortunately, I have yet to attain her level of enlightenment. So instead I'm
just a mere mortal, a pathetic pleb, and I can't let go of the interaction. Even the *idea*
of relinquishing my corporate armor scares me. I've lived under both its weight and
its protection for so long that the thought of being stripped of it feels frightening instead of liberating, as though I'd be left naked and vulnerable.

I know—I distinctly *remember*—a time when I didn't give one tiny shit about
the corporate ladder. But at some point, as I toiled away to pay the bills and make
ends meet, I'd segued from, "This is bullshit, but I do it to eat and pay student loans
and rent," to getting swept up in the rush of advancement and the enjoyment of financial security.

And I'm only 30 and at the director level. How much stickier does the quicksand get the further in you wade? The longer you stay, the higher you climb, and the
more inextricably you weave yourself into a life you don't believe in. At what point,
if ever, do you know that this will be your life...you bought the ticket and the ride
ain't gonna let you off 'til it's done?

I can't be sure when it is. But, unfortunately, I have a sinking feeling that that
point is far behind me.

Chapter Twenty-One

The Nutritional Deficiencies of Corporate Life

The Lowly Needs of Mortals

If I had hoped that my work-life would improve with the twirling departure of my theater-loving, show tunes-singing, wine-guzzling, paranoid, delusional boss… well then, those hopes are quickly dashed. Shortly after Vicky's departure, Charles unexpectedly announces his retirement, and in the ensuing shake-up, Investorcap decides to merge the institutional and personal wealth management marketing departments, the upshot of which is that I will report to none other than Tammy Medusa, my ass-kissing, woman-hating, company champion counterpart from the summit at Beaver Creek.

With a pit in my stomach, I make the requisite call to tell her how delighted I am with this turn of events. "Oh, me too," she says insincerely. "We're thrilled to have you on the team."

I perk up. "Great. I can't wait to meet them. Uh…who's actually on the team?

"Uh…well, the uh…receptionist answers my phone, so it's pretty much like I have an assistant. And now you."

I slump. If I tried to find a silver lining, there would be none. In no uncertain terms, this is the career equivalent of boarding the express train to Armageddon.

Being assigned to report to someone in *personal wealth management* is made even more ridiculous by the fact that Medusa is only my peer in title and has absolutely no experience in institutional asset management *or* public relations. The only thing she did appear to have experience in was kissing senior-management ass and sending emails at three in the morning. Given these habits, my work-life balance was probably not going to improve.

I set my intention to brace up, as Nana says, and make even *this* work. Deeply entrenched in the disaster that surely awaits this ill-advised department merger, I commit to smiling and toiling away no matter what the level of dysfunction. I'm a professional, successful woman. There's no other option.

Vicky's job responsibilities fall to me, which is standard in the corporate world when departures occur without a replacement. Equally standard when stepping up to take over the responsibilities of one's boss is that a corresponding step-up in title and compensation is most definitely *not* included. The strategy seems to be to work the nonexecutives as long and hard as possible without additional compensation and reallocate this savings to the upper echelon's bonus pool.

The effects of these changes start to take a greater toll on my ever-dwindling slice of nonwork life, and most of all, the Nunnally slice. The increase in workload eats into what little time and energy exists outside of our respective careers. There simply isn't enough to go around…and there certainly isn't enough for me.

But because I'm cursed with that innate female desire to do well and please others, I do it. With a smile. Without complaining.

Nunnally tells me to quit, but I ignore him and seek refuge in productivity. Productivity is a place where you can hide for many years. Productivity is the junk food of career satisfaction—it makes you feel full, but nutritionally, it doesn't provide what you need.

Friday arrives and my class files in for the last time. After completing this workshop, the final hurdles between me and the finish line are 40 hours of assisting Thea's classes and finishing my individual project.

Almost everyone heads for wall spaces, wise now, knowing that the back grows quickly weary and you'll be even more sore come Sunday night if you don't claim one of these coveted spots. Only the latecomers are stuck with the unsupported seats. Well, the latecomers and Brinley, of course. She continues to stake out a spot as close as yogically possible to Thea. What's back support compared to proximity to greatness?

Gloria comes in late, doesn't seem to notice that, as has been customary for the past year, everyone is sitting in a giant circle. She sits down *inside* the circle, directly in front of Jessica. Jessica peers around her, first to the left, then to the right, waiting for Gloria to notice. Jessica clears her throat.

Gloria, still oblivious, tousles her hair and looks around smiling. "*Namaste,* everyone! Hello! Hello! *Namaste!*"

After a long moment and no response, Jessica relocates her bolster and blanket perch to the left.

Summer digs some sort of cruciferous vegetable out of her hemp bag.

Annnnd, we're back.

We chant as a group. Everyone knows the mysterious Sanskrit sounds and melody now. The notes and rhythm are second nature. Thea hands out workbooks that are miraculously free of mistakes—tangible proof that it's the end of an era.

"So…our last workshop," Thea says. "Many of you are going into teaching. In terms of readiness, well, you just have to leap into the abyss. It's scary, I know," she admits. "I felt like I was going to vomit when I taught my first class. And that lasted for at least a month!"

We all laugh sympathetically. It's good to feel unified with the group on something. It's also reassuring to see this human side of Thea, which she usually keeps safely behind her strong boundaries.

"There's really no way to prepare. You *will* be nervous. You *will* feel naked and not ready. But you just have to do it—jump off the top of the building. As an adult, it's hard to feel unsure. We want to fix it. Take more workshops. Prepare somehow. But what you really need to do is just let it be. You guys have all the ingredients to teach. Now it's about diving in and letting that be okay. Listen—life is messy. Your first few classes will be messy. Let them be!"

I'm not even going to teach, but I tighten my ponytail reflexively at the mention of "messy," then force my fingers to release. Once again, it occurs to me that Thea is talking about a concept that could be useful off the mat as well.

"If you're so busy criticizing yourself and agonizing over your shortcomings, you'll miss what your *students* are actually doing—the mistakes they're making. We need to be willing to be less than efficient and perfect. Just be patient. Be willing to be seen as human and humble. Show humility in your imperfection."

I sit back and admire her. Thea's on point and insightful. Is the core of my desire for neatness and efficiency really a desire for perfection? If so, I know logically that I'm setting myself up to fail. Thea's counsel to allow ourselves to be seen as fallible requires a lot of courage. And is exactly right.

"It's healing and helpful to your students to see that you're not perfect. If you wait until you're perfect to go out as teachers, your students aren't going to be able to connect to you or learn from you. Who can connect with perfection?"

This concept also rings true. Thea's honesty about her own teaching anxiety is tremendously reassuring. In fact, she's never seemed more reachable. And as a result, I feel more connected to her and what she's saying. I wonder what it would be like if she did this more often. Feeling all yoga-ey and wise, I wonder what others miss out on when I hide the cracks in my personal and professional facades. What if I dropped those facades?

Instantly, the yogic vibe vanishes. My jaw clenches at the thought of being so vulnerable at the office. In front of the corporate barracudas? They'd jump on those perceived weaknesses so fast, my head would spin. It would be like a flock of buzzards landing on a badly battered but still-live kill. Before I could defend myself, they'd dig their beaks into the cracks until I finally gave up and died.

Professionally, it's not an option, but the fact that I live a life of constant pretense and image projection gives me food for thought.

"Let us consider the themes of service and insight," Thea says, first thing Saturday morning as we prepare for our final weekend of assisting her semi-private therapeutic sessions. "We'll be seeing clients with everything from depression to spinal injuries. Remember that each body is unique. We need to share our deeply authentic appreciation for our clients' uniquenesses. Create a space free from judgment. Reinforce this with your essence and your language. Nourish your students by demonstrating self-acceptance. Heal and harmonize by embracing each one's highest potential. Forget the yoga norm."

I write this down.

I remember back to my first day of the immersion: only a handful of the women had stereotypical "yoga bodies"—the kind of body that female celebrities famously claim they derive from their yoga practices but later are revealed to be derived from a coke habit, with an eating disorder and a prescription-pill "practice" on the side. Feeling safe and a sense of compassion are the essence of Thea's teaching. These are traits I admire.

"As adults, we forget to appreciate the beauty and perfection of imperfection. But as teachers, we need to resist this temptation. Okay, now let's get started because I want to make sure you have a lunch break today…I know Sara *needs* to eat!"

My head jerks up at the unanticipated dig. My face turns beet red. I want to retreat into a ball of shame, but decide I won't let it slide. "I'm sure other people want to eat lunch and have a break too," I say.

"Well, everybody gets hungry, but I know you *really* need to eat," Thea says.

And that is one thing I won't miss—feeling like a loser for being a mere mortal. Not to mention getting called out on it in front of the group.

It's emotional whiplash that this comes on the heels of those good feelings Thea evoked in showing her humanity and really connecting with us. These events stand in stark contrast. On the one hand are Thea's obvious strengths as an incredibly talented teacher and, when she chooses, a real ability to open up and connect, but on the other are her aloofness and patronizing comments. But is this so different from anyone? Don't we all have our contradictions? More food for thought as the first round of clients stream in.

The rest of the weekend passes in a blur of observing intakes and assisting clients in their therapeutic sequences. On Sunday, the last day of the training, we actually get a real lunch break. Pointedly, Thea has ensured that today we'll have the whole hour. Whether that is due to my ignoble need to eat or an improvement in her time-management skills, I don't know, but I'll take it.

Jessica and I head outside. As we walk past an unused studio, we see the rest of our classmates gathered inside. Immediately, my heart clutches—is this another coup? "What do you think that's about?" I ask Jessica.

"Who knows?" Jessica laughs. "I'm sure it has nothing to do with you. They're probably drawing straws to see who gets to sit closest to Thea this afternoon."

"Or who gets to bring her afternoon herbal tea?" I suggest.

"Or who will be her fave next week," Jessica adds.

We head toward the car, but I can't shake the feeling that I'm getting ganged up on again.

Lunch in a public setting, away from the training and all it entails, is, as always, a welcome and wonderful break. My clenched brain, which has basically assumed the fetal position after the repeated pummeling of taking in copious amounts of new information in compressed amounts of time, unwinds just a bit. Jessica and I chat about vital, life-changing topics like the new avocado-green bag she found at the Freeport outlets and how I've never been to Maine and really want to see a moose.

Jessica assures me I won't see one near the outlets in Freeport.

I glance at my watch. "Time to go back," I say. It seems far too soon.

As we return, we see the same cluster of trainees in the unused studio. This time, there's even more activity and chatter.

Jessica and I pointedly make eye contact and, without a word, walk in.

We hover awkwardly on the peripheries of the circle. "Hey guys, what's up?" I ask, feeling painfully like a sixth-grade girl approaching the knot of boys at a school dance.

Joyce, one of the long-distance students who I'd never gotten to know, answers. "Oh...hey." Her eyes slide away from us guiltily. "We...uh...decided to buy Thea a thank-you gift. You know, for training all of us." She gestures to the hardcover book in her hands. "She's been wanting this one."

There is a long, awkward pause while I wonder *how* she knew that since Thea never reveals a single personal thing about herself. It then occurs to me that some planning had gone into this, and that Jessica and I, at least, were left out.

Jessica and I look at each other. She's clearly thinking the same thing.

"Oh." I pause, waiting for Joyce to offer to include us in the gift. She doesn't. "Well, is this just from you? Or from our whole class?"

"No, no. It's from our whole class...from all of us." Joyce gestures to the whole group. The question of how it can be from "all of us" when not "all" of us knew about it hovers unasked.

"Okay. Well, what do I owe you for it?" I plunge back in, awkward but determined to be included or die trying.

"Yeah, I'll throw some money in too," Jessica echoes.

"Oh, there's really no need," Joyce assures us breezily.

Jessica and I exchange another look.

"I'm happy to," I say.

"Me too," Jessica adds. "Just let us know how much."

Joyce is smiling kindly but with that same sense of impenetrability that Thea exudes. "Oh. Well, okay. Whatever you're comfortable contributing is fine."

I'm getting irritated. Even for math-challenged me, this is a simple calculation: price of the book divided by number of students. "Well, how much was the book?"

"Honestly, whatever you're comfortable with is fine," Joyce insists.

Jessica reaches for her purse.

"Well...are you the one who bought it?" I press.

230

She nods.

"So…how much was it?" *And why are you making me drag this out of you, you bogi?*

"Twenty-five," she admits reluctantly.

"Well, I have a five," Jessica says, handing her a bill.

"Whatever you're comfortable with," Joyce reiterates.

Thoroughly annoyed, I give her the same. But if more than five of us did this, Joyce recouped the modest cost of the book and is now profiting. Not that any of it really matters.

"There's also a card Jaznae picked out if you'd like to sign it. We're giving it with the book," Joyce adds reluctantly as she takes the money.

We head toward Jaznae, who is perched royally on a bolster, supervising as Summer draws an elaborate drum doodle next to her name.

I add my name to the card, while still not feeling any more included. Unintentionally, this is the most fitting end to this year. This time, however, I'm totally okay with the feeling of exclusion.

Back in session a few minutes later, our class forms a seated circle for the last time. Jaznae, Joyce, and Brinley ceremoniously march up to Thea. "A token of our appreciation for guiding our evolution and our journey," Joyce says.

Thea smiles widely, but nods as though she's been expecting this. She takes the gifts. "Oh," she says still smiling, looking down at the book. "Oh." She opens the card next, "Isn't that funny? Last year's class got me this exact same card."

The rest of the group giggles; karma is a silly goose.

Thea sets the card and book aside and asks if there are any final questions. The possibility of a graduation dinner is raised. Instantaneously, innumerable dietary constraints come pouring forth.

"I'm a vegetarian, but not a vegan…."

"I'm trying to be free of judgment—but as a vegan practicing *ahimsa*, I can on-ly go somewhere vegan!"

"I'm avoiding gluten...."

"I'm merging the Judaism of my family of origin and my emerging Hinduism through yoga, so I'd like a kosher Indian place...."

"I'm only eating raw foods this year!"

"Sorry. I can't eat anything raw."

"As yogis, we believe we'll nourish ourselves on the many levels of our beings by eating at *ayurvedically* recommended times. That means six pm exactly."

"Since The Birth, I'm on Persephone's schedule, so I'll need to play the time by ear. It would feel inauthentic to try to commit to a time I may not be able to actu-ally attend."

I consider recommending a group trip to the lost city of Atlantis. But I also know, after a year with these folks, that even if such a restaurant could be found, the plan will never actually happen because this roomful of yogis isn't capable of coor-dinating and executing a dinner where everyone shows up at the same place, at the same time, on the same night.

After deciding to "meditate about it, then correspond by email"—yoga code for "ain't never gonna happen"—we chant a final time. The room erupts in hugs and promises to stay in touch. I avoid Janet and Jaznae.

To my surprise, Thea approaches me. "Have you considered the *Seva* Rotation?"

I flash back to the immersion, when Thea had announced the *Seva* Rotation, eliciting a veritable yoga stampede. I'd happily stepped aside. It had never occurred to me that I could be a chosen one. An ungraceful, disbelieving snort escapes me. "Me?"

She is smiling, encouraging, nodding. "You should! I think it would be a good fit."

"*Me?*" I echo again, like a complete moron. Me who "really needs" lunch breaks? Who "runs away" from her problems doing cardio? Who got kicked out of

232

her own group? Who has "relational issues" to chaos? *Me*? Not Brinley—Thea's constant shadow? Not any of the others who'd vied for her attention and sprinted to agree with her every fleeting thought? Not Joyce who'd gone to the trouble of procuring the mysterious book for her? Then again, there were three *Seva* spots available. I had no idea who the others would go to. It didn't matter. I was among the chosen! I couldn't believe it!

"I think you're ready and it would be great for you. You have the tools, Sara. You have the knowledge. You're ready Think about it." Then, just as suddenly, as though I'm usurping too much of her time, she walks away.

As I drive home, I reflect on the weekend. In the client sessions, I'd helped people whose various injuries and limitations had run the gamut from severe scoliosis to depression and anxiety. Propping and assisting them around these issues had been like doing a jigsaw puzzle—I'd worked to fit each pose around the unique shape of their needs or constraints. And, like a puzzle, it had been both challenging and rewarding to make yoga accessible to them.

It was also a new way of thinking. For as long as I'd been practicing, I'd thought of yoga as something physical. From my first class in the sweaty gym basement, it was a way to burn off the searing pain of a broken heart; newly defined arm muscles and a calmer mind were welcome byproducts. Beyond that, I hadn't stopped to consider what yoga was or why I felt better after I did it.

But after seeing such a variety of clients this weekend, I now realize that the practice of yoga itself is pliant and flexible. And the benefits of the practice go far deeper than strength and flexibility—they stretch to students cultivating compassion toward themselves.

With this newfound awareness, I recognize that my appreciation of yoga is evolving. Somewhere along the way, my old, striving power yoga classes had stopped feeling good. I left them feeling wanting, unsatisfied—like when I get stuck working and don't get to take a lunch break and then, hours later, on the brink of a complete meltdown/hunger-induced crying jag, inhale an entire bag of microwave popcorn and feel full, but not really *fed* afterward.

Well, at least now I know: popcorn doesn't cut it—on the mat or off.

Chapter Twenty-Two

The Last Hurrah of Corporate Life

Prototypical Behavior of the Female Barracuda

A few weeks later, an emergency company-wide meeting is called. The CEO announces he's resigning to accept another position. This abrupt departure clearly indicates that the company will be going through a major reorganization. From a personal standpoint, this is more bad news. As the head of PR, I've handled CEO hirings, firings, and desertions many times before—but always with advance notice.

What a nightmare! I think, as I stand with 90 of my colleagues, trying to absorb this news. *I can't believe that they're telling me this now! I should've been in on this weeks ago! Silly corporate morons. When will they learn?* Frantically, I begin scribbling random notes in no particular order: *shape messaging, contact media, write company statement, issue press release, write internal announcement, write external announcement*....

"We've been working on this for the past week," the CEO says, "with PR help from Tammy."

I freeze. The consequence of his words sinks slowly into my brain. *Tammy Medusa?* The slave-driving woman-hating, ass-kissing middle manager who'd recently become my boss? She's in the Midwest! I'm suddenly cold even as my cheeks turn hot. *Medusa? Handling PR?* My brain scrambles...*wait...that's my job! Or...*was *my job.*

My brain spirals around like a speeding car on a patch of ice. *Is this actually happening? Was it just announced—in front of everyone—that my peer, my new "boss," is now doing my job? My new boss who has no experience in or knowledge of public relations or institutional money management?* The careening car that is my brain lurches off the road, flips over, and lands in a ditch. It seizes and then stops altogether. My hearts seems to stop with it. I look around frantically, desperate to run away.

"Isn't that your job?" a voice beside me quietly asks. I turn. It's Betsy.

I nod dumbly. Anxiety rushes over me. I'm helpless. Cornered. Lost.

What feels like a thousand eyes turn to look at me, then back to the CEO as he describes "Tammy's excellent PR efforts."

The surrealistic contradiction of time both decelerating so that everyone and everything around me seems to be in slow motion, yet speeding up so that mentally I've already leapt ahead to what this means and how I can escape—combines to create a brain-twizzling scramble. My knees buckle. I might faint. If I do, please let it be graceful.

Someone, Betsy I think, puts an arm around me and says something comforting. But my pulse is thundering so loudly in my ears that I don't hear her. I can't see through my utter humiliation. I'm sweating profusely and hoping she won't notice. I command myself not to cry. *Don't you dare! Don't. You. Fucking. Dare.*

Medusa—evidently no longer in the Midwest and apparently the new me— steps to the front and begins offering up the usual obligatory prattle. "It's an honor to be a part of this team...I couldn't have done it without the support of senior management...I was planning to fly back to Podunk tonight but of course I can stay and work through the weekend...happy to...work first, always work first...."

I edge shakily toward the door. Blindly, I rush back to my office. I pull random stuff—lipstick, a bag of almonds, a birthday card I'd forgotten to send—out of drawers and stuff it all into my bag.

I've never been so completely embarrassed in my entire life.

I call Nunnally compulsively. Each call goes to voicemail. My throat is tight. It burns. I can barely breathe. *I'm leaving! No! I'm going to stomp down to HR and tell this company to go screw themselves!*

There's a sharp rap on my door. I look up to see Medusa herself. She enters without permission. The walls of my office suction in. It's suddenly too small in here. She's too close. I scramble backwards in my expensive wheelie chair. I rise awkwardly. Stand so I don't have to look up at her. It doesn't matter. She's triumphant; a tiny smirk bares her fanglike teeth. "I've been over in the Marriot for a week. But it's much better to be here. No more hiding."

I try to absorb that. *So that's how she managed to pull this off—lurking unseen as she waited to attack. Corporate barracuda in a cheap suit.*

According to a special I'd seen once, barracudas are opportunistic, insatiable predators. Fearsome enemies, they rely on surprise and speed to overtake their victims. Barracudas are sometimes known to prey on fish as large as themselves. They attack viciously—skewering their victims and often even slicing them in half.

And that's exactly what Medusa had done. And now she'd come to gloat. She looks as happy as I've ever seen her—amped up, I can only imagine, on adrenaline and victory.

Purposely, she leaves the door open, relishing an audience. And she has one—curious co-workers rubberneck to watch what's unfolding as they leave the meeting. Medusa barely manages to restrain herself from cackling gleefully. "We have a lot to do. I'll be needing your help for the rest of the day to manage the PR." Her voice is carefully measured, matter of fact, condescending. She might as well have said, "Fetch me coffee, bitch."

Rage kicks in. "Oh? It seems you've 'managed' things so far on your own," I choke out—barely—disgust tingeing my words. If this was a movie, I'd fly at her neck like a spider monkey.

She ignores that. "I need you to put together lists of everyone we need to notify."

I'm just about to tell her that if she doesn't know how to do this job, maybe she shouldn't have taken it, when my phone rings. I see Nunnally's number. "Excuse me, this is urgent."

"Well, *this* is urgent, and we need to start working." She's getting snarkier and more hostile by the syllable.

"I'll be with you shortly." I turn away. "This is Sara," I say into the phone, by way of cutting her off.

Reluctantly, she leaves, pointing to her watch as she goes.

"What the hell is going on?" Nunnally demands, concern laced with panic in his voice. "I have 20 missed calls from you!"

I choke out the news, holding the phone to my ear as I shimmy around my desk as far as the cord will stretch and nudge the door shut with the tip of one shoe. *Wait. Is this me? Am I saying this? Is this really happening?* The door clicks shut. I fall heavily in my chair, shaking.

"*What?*"

I wrangle a last, desperate attempt to hold it together. I bite my lip until it hurts, trying to get control of myself at least, if not this situation. But it's futile. Like seams ripping open, a gasp wrests free of my control, and tears race down my face faster than I knew tears could go. I fold in half, pressing my elbows on my knees. Through the glass office walls—a symbol of Investorcap's openness and transparency, ha!—I hope it looks as though I'm searching for something under my desk. An earring? A pen? I can't breathe or speak. My body is heaving. I choke on my own snot. I clutch the phone with one hand and my forehead with the other.

Nunnally's voice sets intractably. "After all you've done for them? Hell, no!" Nunnally, the kindest, most patient, most tolerant person I've ever met is pissed. *Really pissed.* It feels good. "You need to go down to HR and tell them they can take this job and shove it up their ass." His anger is a protective shield. I cower behind it.

The thought is too terrifying. I've never been good at standing up to bullies. "I can't."

"Yes you can—and you have to. Now get down there and tell them you're finished. Effective immediately."

I take a deep, shaky breath and make myself hang up. I feel like a fighter who's been knocked down—flat on my back, the wind sucked out of my lungs by some bigger force. I'm lying there, breathless and stunned, lacerated and smarting, internally battered and externally bleeding, but there is still another round to go before I can crawl out of the ring. I have to get up and finish this. The thought isn't an appealing one, but I can do it.

I put my head between my knees. When I've steadied my breathing, I straighten up. I twist my hair into an even-tighter bun. Apply lipstick. Put on my suit jacket. Stride directly past the guest office Medusa has commandeered and down to HR before I lose my nerve.

"Sara, can't this wait?" the short-haired secretary that I usually have a very collegial relationship with asks impatiently. "Today's not a good day."

"No, it really *can't*." Something in my tone indicates I won't be moved or placated.

She ushers me in to the head of HR's office. I haven't seen her since I reported Vicky, but nothing has changed. Today her cowboy boots are turquoise. Presumably to accent her dangly silver and turquoise earrings.

"What can I do for you, darlin'?" she asks in a way that only a Texan can. She's a caricature of herself. It fits this situation.

I sit down. In a perversely calm post-traumatic way, I outline the innumerable ways I have "added value" over the years. I refresh her memory about Vomiting Vicky's antics, my current reassignment to utterly unqualified Medusa, and, to top off this glorious run, how my new boss had just taken over my job. Publicly.

I outline the scandals I'd managed, crises I'd averted, and the proverbial bombs I'd disarmed. And through it all, I'd smiled and worked harder. I'd sacrificed my energy, personal time, relationships, marriage, and, you know, that triviality sometimes called a life outside of work.

I explain all this to the head of HR, who smiles and nods and makes understanding clucking noises that lead me to believe—almost—that she understands where I'm coming from and is, perhaps, on my side.

However, I tell her, even I have my limit and by God, when I've reached it, That. Is. It. I take a deep breath and lay it out for her. "There is only so much shit I'll eat before I'm done eating shit, and today I AM DONE EATING SHIT!"

She continues leaning back in her chair, one substantial ankle resting on the other sizable knee. She nods congenially.

My stomach clenches. "Consider this my official resignation. I won't be finishing out the day." This is both a lie and a bluff. Of course I'm going to finish out the day. I'm a stick-to-it freak who can never let anything go. I'm a professional, dammit.

I wait for her to beg me to stay. To offer me anything. Instead, she says, "Sara, I'm very sorry to hear that that's the way you feel. Are you sure you don't want to take a little more time to think this over?" Her manner is calm and perfunctory.

"I'm sure," I say, even though I'm not.

"Of course," she nods. "I'll take care of the appropriate notifications, and we'll have operations bring some boxes to your office for you to pack up your personal effects."

I unclip my company ID. I place it photo side up on her desk. There I am, beaming with hope way back on my first day. It's scratched and the photo is faded now. I slide it over to her. The nagging fear of being denied entry at the security turnstiles is official. I won't be able to get in.

Just like that, it's done.

And that's when I realize that all my sacrifices and work mean nothing to this company. This cold, uncaring corporation doesn't give one tiny shit about me. I think of the holiday weekends I've worked through. I think of late nights at the office distractedly slurping up bad pizza with my colleagues instead of meals with Nunnally…or family…or friends. I think of all the events I'd missed because it hadn't seemed possible to take time off from work. I think about the fact that, aside from our honeymoon, I haven't taken a vacation in over five years because there's always so much work. How I haven't been home for a holiday because I just can't bear the idea of more travel. Tears sting the backs of my eyes and I shrink into myself. My chest collapses like a deflating balloon. It was all for nothing. It was all for a job I don't have anymore.

I return to my office on wobbly legs. I cram as many personal items (wedding picture, yoga mat, spare shoes, samples of my work) into my commuting bag as possible. In this industry, it's customary to be escorted out by security. I won't have the chance to come back for anything. I throw everything else into the boxes that are brought to my office and address them to myself.

As I walk past Medusa's office, I keep my eyes straight ahead. I fantasize fleetingly of telling her I hope she chokes on her success as she devours my job, but I won't give her the satisfaction of a scene.

I take the elevators down 40 floors for the last time. The doors ping open. My heels click-click through the marble lobby. It's relatively empty by now. I walk woodenly through the revolving doors, out into the daylight, and traipse slowly home.

The apartment is eerily quiet. I feel like a trespasser. *What are you doing here at this time?* The clock asks with each tick. I drop my bags unceremoniously in the middle of the floor and dissolve into tears on the couch. I couldn't care less that my crisp suit is wrinkling.

It's a surreal experience to be forced to leave a job you hate. You'd think that I'd feel sheer, unadulterated relief, followed by joy. A sense of freedom. And that will probably come. But first there is this overwhelming and infuriating sense of powerlessness.

I feel *enraged* and yet impotent—as though I don't have the ability to control my own life. Choice and control have been seized from me. Like a child whose chore has been taken away from her—the ultimate indignity—I feel an overwhelming sense of shame, failure, and deep-down resentment.

As a modern-day woman, I'm used to—no, I *thrive* on—controlling every controllable aspect of my life. I'd always felt I was at the helm of my own destiny. I'd risen to the professional level that I had, not on connections or luck, but under my own steam. I'd taken pride in my professional accomplishments.

Because I hadn't believed in or loved my job, I had learned to make it bearable by deriving satisfaction and pride in what I could accomplish within it. I had launched a PR program. Built it from the ground up. Grown it into the powerful program it currently was. Made it successful, garnering appearances in the crown jewels of the media world. I'd been nominated two years running for the Most Valuable

Employee award. I had made a difference—*a significant difference, damn it*—to this company.

So why hadn't they valued me and my work? Why hadn't they protected me against this latest installment of crazy? *Why…?*

That I didn't care one whit about what the company did and that it unequivocally didn't make a positive impact on the world haunted me, but I'd quieted those bothersome qualms by focusing on what the job had enabled me to do: repay my student loans, buy a condo, make car payments, etc. There was value in that, especially to me. Having grown up poor, I knew well the keen sharpness of scarcity, never having nice things, and always struggling to make do. This career path had allowed me the luxury of escaping that misery. I had never intended to invest a decade of my life into this soulless existence. But since I had, I wanted to stay and succeed.

Now even that has been taken from me.

I wish I'd screamed at Medusa, "You can't get rid of me, *I quit!*"

I wish I'd made the break years ago. How dare they let some unqualified asskisser take over my job! How dare they belittle me and the work I had done that way!

Eventually, my rage turns toward myself—what had I been thinking to waste a decade in an industry I hated? Why hadn't I listened to that little voice that had whispered, then spoken, then lectured, then shouted, to quit years ago? When I was 22…25…29…30? With every year, every raise, every title boost, and every perk (like the undeniable allure of having an office *with a door*, first-class corporate travel, and extravagant dinners out at fancy restaurants…unless I was with the pennypincher in New Jersey)…and the ear of the C-level execs who ran the company…and respect…and status…and visibility…with each tiny advancement, it had become harder and harder to walk away.

As I had gotten further away from the financial struggles I'd grown up with, as I experienced the ease of buying not just the heavily discounted items—be it pasta (so what if it wasn't the kind I wanted?) or work clothes (who cared if the only size they had left was too small? I'd lose a few pounds or leave the jacket unbuttoned!)—

the comfort became addictive. The advancement became addictive. Then I blinked, and ten years had gone by working in this industry. And now that very industry that I disdained had let me walk without a word of protest like I was nothing to them.

It was entirely too reminiscent of getting laid off from my first finance job after getting dumped by my post-college boyfriend. I'd learned my lesson in the relationship department, but had kept returning to the same burning barn for far too many years in the career category. And, just like any bad relationship that ends in inevitable devastation, I was mad at them for doing it and doubly mad at myself for staying long enough to let them. Damn them and damn me for my own damn stupidity.

The afternoon passes torturously as I wait for Nunnally to come home and give me a hug. As usual, he's stuck working late...because his firm still values him, dammit. So I sit alone and cry angry, humiliated, self-pitying tears. Anxiety, fueled by uncertainty and fear, sweeps in. What will the future hold? Where am I going?

And last—perhaps scariest of all—isn't this what I'd wanted for a long, long time?

Part Three:

I'm a Yoga Teacher...Now What?

Chapter Twenty-Three
No Job? No Stress? But What Do I Do?

On my first day of not working, I'm determined to start a new schedule. I'll go for a run in the morning! I'll eat cupcakes for breakfast! I'll read a book…for fun! I'll even sleep in! On a Monday! Just because I can. Because I'm jobless. Because I'm now a bad-ass, anti-corporate rebel!

Of course, this is not to be. My eyes zing open at exactly, to the minute, when my alarm should go off. Long accustomed to the corporate schedule, I don't even need the intrusive beeping anymore. I close my eyes to try to fight off consciousness. I will myself to succumb to the welcoming womb of slumber. I'm a bad-ass, anti-corporate rebel. By God, I! Will! Sleep! In!

But I can't.

Nunnally leaves for work. Outside, the street starts to buzz with the corporate commute and then everyone gets to their desks and it subsides. As the neighborhood lapses into its own midmorning lull, it occurs to me that I know little about its rhythms, but I know the office's rhythms by heart. Angela would be finishing her Dunkin' Donuts skim coffee and looking for stilettos on sale at Neiman's. Betsy would be answering four incessantly ringing lines, checking celebrity gossip sites, and chucking dried mango slices at me. The Meat and the sales guys would be surreptitiously surfing for porn, talking about the noteworthy body parts of female colleagues, or reliving the big weekend game.

I should be at my desk, having my morning coffee and getting into my day, phone lines ringing and emails pinging incessantly. A creature who dearly loves familiarity, I'd enjoyed the comforting predictability of the morning office bustle for years. It had felt like home. Now at my actual home, solitary and routineless, I feel weirdly out of place. For so long, I'd chafed under the bonds of my corporate life, but now I missed them. It is those very tasks that provided the direction and structure that marshaled my days. They were the anchor and the lighthouse of my daily life. Without their constraints, and also their purpose, I feel untethered and rudderless.

Despite feeling as though I'd tumbled down a rabbit hole to a foreign world— and acutely aware of the irony that this foreign world is actually my home—some things remain the same. Nana still calls my cell phone at exactly 9:00 am to remind me to look both ways before crossing and to see what I've got planned for the day. She, at least, doesn't seem to mind that I'm not at work. She's still basking in her inordinate relief that I'm finally married.

Unfortunately, I'm not as calm. I'm freaking out and don't know what to do with myself. I wander, aimless and terrified, around the apartment, which is steeped in a strange early morning quiet.

As I stand awkwardly in the middle of the living room, my cell rings again. It's the chief economist at one of our partner companies. Apparently, she's going to be attending a series of press conferences throughout Southeast Asia, culminating in India. She wants me to go as her personal PR rep.

I can't believe it! A free, first-class trip around the world, ending in India! For-get Bachelor's Gulch, New Jersey, and all the other equally unmemorable trips. This was Southeast Asia! And most important, *India*—a place I'd dreamed of going ever since I was old enough to watch the Discovery Channel. The idea that one country could boast everything from the lithe majesty of Asiatic lions to the quiet, dignified enormity of elephants, and *also* gestate the roots of yoga, was almost too much. If it wouldn't affect my yoga balance, I would've considered sacrificing my right pinky toe in order to go. And now, here it was—this wonderful, golden opportunity. All expenses paid. No pinky-toe sacrifice required. Krishna smiled on my fortunes! Karma loved me! *Ganesha*, the elephant god, remover of obstacles, was paving the way to yoga Graceland!

Then I remember why I'm in our living room instead of at the office. I swallow hard and tell her I resigned on Friday. She'll have to take Medusa instead. The words feel like vomiting up shards of glass followed by a shot of vinegar and a side of stomach acid.

With that ironic start to my day, I realize I have to settle in. I look around our place. It's cluttered and unkempt. Usually, neither Nunnally nor I has time to deal with it. Laundry stays heaped in the hamper until we run out of socks or underwear. Dry cleaning doesn't go out until we have no more shirts to wear. Dishes aren't done because they're mostly unused—neither of us has time to buy or prepare food. Our engagement picture sits rolled up against a wall because neither of us has found time to frame or hang it. Our winter and summer clothes, which are rotated out of necessity (no space in city living) to an inaccessible storage loft in the bedroom that you need a ladder to get to, haven't been rotated. So we're still in wool despite it being May.

Conversely, we keep our suitcases handy as we both travel so frequently there's absolutely no point in bothering to go through the hassle of getting out the ladder and stashing them in the loft, only to climb up again a few days later when we're back on the road. Our front doorknob hasn't worked since we moved in, but we haven't had time to find or hire a repairman. And even if we had, neither of us could've stayed home from work while it was fixed. Ditto with the grouting around the bathtub. Instead of a home, it feels like a transit station. We live at work or on the road. This is just somewhere we stop in before we take off again.

Resignedly, I try to tackle the cleaning, but there is so much to be done that the task seems endless —sort of like trying to empty a swimming pool with an eyedropper. I decide to go food shopping and spend over $200 on replenishing basics. I try to make dinner, but I can't think of anything except spaghetti with canned red sauce, which is our standby when we do eat at home. I know there was a time when I had loved to cook, but I can't remember what.

The day wears on. The sensation of being rudderless and disoriented grows.

I plummet into a pit of worry. What's going to happen with my career? How will I explain my abrupt departure to prospective employers? What will my next job be anyway? Should I stay in PR? Am I doing that because it's the right career for me or because it's what I know how to do? What else am I qualified to do?

Well, I am *qualified to teach yoga,* I think to myself. Maybe I should leverage this as a natural opportunity to give it a try. I had just invested thousands of dollars and a year of my life into teacher training. But, aside from my run-in with Taxerina and subsequently wondering how our conversation might've gone differently if I'd had to introduce myself as a yoga teacher instead of as the Director of Public Relations at Investorcap, I had never considered teaching.

Teaching always seemed like it was for impractical bubbleheads who weren't firmly rooted in reality. Who didn't have mortgages and students loans. Who thought that shaving and deodorant were optional, but bell-bottoms, hemp, and tie-dye were necessities. Who didn't give a rat's patootie about responsibilities, punctuality, deadlines, or efficiency—the mainstays of my existence.

Then again, I'd just invested a lot of time, energy, and money into deepening my knowledge of yoga. Maybe it was time to put it to use instead of simply having my now-deeper practice continue serve as life support for a never-ending existence within the corporate world. *Still though...a career in yoga?* It seems ludicrous. But I guess I could see if the hemp and bell-bottoms fit, then make a choice between corporate work and yoga.

The visceral shudder that occurs deep down in my gut at the thought of returning to corporate life signals that that option isn't a great idea.

With all these questions whirling around my brain, and a cloud of uncertainty hanging on me like bad perfume, I decide to take a class with Thea on Day Two of Not Working.

I arrive in the familiar, candlelit room with the illuminated Buddha at the front, claim a spot near the wall, and reverently roll out my mat. I sit in *sukhasana,* easy pose, and begin *ujjiy* breathing. I'm determined to shut off my brain and its incessant questions. But it's impossible.

What's my next job going to be? How long will it take me to get it? If only I knew, I could relax. Maybe I should have waited to quit until I lined up something else. Was that really stupid? Will I end up with a gap in my resume? Maybe I should try to do some consulting right away...or...oh just SHUT UP! STOP WORRYING! Oh crap. I wonder if I worry too much. Maybe I have an actual anxiety disorder. Maybe I should look into that. Or maybe I should just get a real job so that I don't have to worry about it. Or maybe I should take a little time off. But I can't enjoy it because I'm so freaking worried about what's going to happen. God, if my friends knew I was this tortured, they'd really think I was a freak....

Thea enters the room and begins the guided drop-in. I try to still my mind, but thoughts pop up frustratingly like a frenetic game of Whac-A-Mole. *Should an unemployed person really be shelling out 24 bucks for a yoga class? Isn't this a bit wasteful? Oh for God's sake, just stop!*

We emerge from the drop-in and begin breathwork. And for the first time, I notice I start to relax almost immediately in response. My heart flutters at this modest, but telling, success. Thea really is an incredible teacher.

Then, by strange providence or at least eerie coincidence, Thea says, "For this evening's class, we're going to focus on transitions."

A cornerstone of Tri Dosha Yoga is slow, mindful transitions between poses. In general, it's a deliberate, slow, mindful practice. This is in stark contrast to some other types of yoga—such as the *ashtanga* tradition in which I'd started, where speeding through the practice is the norm. In *ashtanga*, the extent of your advancement is more heralded than the work that brought you there, but Tri Dosha Yoga focuses attention on the time and space between poses. I'd known that. I practiced that. It was familiar. However, I'd never been in a class in which the *entire* focus was the transitions. I wonder, again, if this tiny yoga master is a mind reader.

Thea talks about the importance of how we regard transitions. "Are they something to just 'get through'?" she asks as we balance excruciatingly on our right legs, the left thrust high in a standing half-split.

I nod at the truth of this as all the blood rushes to my head.

"Are transitions something we ignore in our rush to 'arrive' at the next pose?" Thea asks, calmly regarding us.

My standing leg feels as though it's on fire. The muscles scream for release and start quivering. As I balance wobbily, a rush of anger surges as Thea keeps talking. She suggests we examine our relationship with transitions. I grit my teeth. *When for the love of God and all that is holy is she going to stop lecturing and get us down? Just finish already!*

As though she finally feels my desperation, she brings the class out of the standing half-split. I slump with relief. Then, as though she'd never felt my desperation at all, she guides us into a low lunge. Still on the right leg. My relief evaporates. I opt out and slip backward into child's pose for a rest. I press my forehead gratefully on the mat. The rest of the class continues in their low lunges before Thea eventually directs them back to child's pose as well.

It's only then that I realize—in a grand mind-zap of irony—that I just altogether skipped a transition. My need to end my discomfort coupled with my predisposition to rush through everything, had won out over Thea's suggestion to focus on transitions. Unfortunately, this isn't the first time.

Why am I always in such an all-fired hurry anyway? What exactly am I trying to get *to*? Some mystical place where I take a good satisfied look around and think, *Yup, I've made it.* Nana would say the final destination is six feet under. No need to rush that. Yet I *do* constantly rush, and in my haste to arrive at the next destination, be it pose or job or appointment or wedding or yoga training or getting home from training, I've been missing the in-between, the middle parts. The *transitions*.

Abruptly, it dawns on me, that life, or at least huge chunks of it, lies in those in-between parts, and in the transformative processes we experience while we're trying to get to wherever we're going.

The excitement over this discovery quickly fades to anxiety. *Oh. My. God. I've been missing my own life!* Would I feel so frantic and anxious all the time if I weren't so busy rushing?

Before I can totally freak out about all the days, hours, heck, *years* I've rushed through to get to—well, who knows what actually—I rein myself in. I have a choice and I can start to make a change now. I take a slow, full breath. I'm not going to waste my 24 bucks or this hour and a half worrying about the *past*.

On my next deep breath, I take another step back from the anxiety cliff as I resolve not to hurry through this transition from Investorcap to—(deepest breath yet)—whatever comes next. I will endeavor to make this transitional time—between jobs, between careers, between stages in my life…just *between*—mindful and deliberate. For once, I resolve, I'm going to let the transition be exactly what it is. Whatever it is.

For the rest of the practice, I keep pulling myself back. Back from worries about the future or regrets about wasted time in the past. Back to the present moment. Back to staying mentally anchored to my practice. It isn't easy, but at least it's a start.

I resolve to carry this commitment off the mat as well.

I commence my transitional phase by creating a home yoga practice. The solitude and self-discipline are challenging, but I make myself unroll the mat every day.

And in the even-less-sexy department, my next effort is learning how to regrout a bathtub. I teach myself to install a new doorknob and lock system, and I try not to mind that it takes me half a day and hours on the phone with customer support. (Yes, they actually have customer support for installing doorknobs. Thank you, lock gods.)

I fix, clean, arrange, and generally shape our house into more of the home I want it to be. I remember how much I love to work with my hands.

I dig out cookbooks we received as wedding gifts but have never used and begin to make dinner every night, thus rediscovering my long-neglected love of cooking. I remember how, many years ago, I loved to simply thumb through recipes, reverently looking at the beautiful photos, reading the ingredient lists like they're sacred texts as I imagined the meals I'd make.

I remember how much I love to disregard the recipe and follow my own instincts for flavor. I think of my Nana as I wear her apron, and of my Aunt Joan—both lovers of great food, and call them for recipes.

My aunt Joan knows the secret brisket recipe and sage wisdom for all of my life's trials and tribulations. Having relied on her my whole life as a mentor, I wonder how I lost the time to call her more often.

When I call Nana to ask her how to make her garlicky roast chicken, she calls me back when it's time to turn it.

And again when it's time to put the potatoes on to boil.

And again when it's time to take everything out of the oven and off the stove.

Nunnally declares me the greatest cook on Earth and himself the luckiest man alive because he gets to eat it all. I start to make notes on the margin of the recipe cards or cookbook pages, creating a food memory trail. I start to feel more fully "fed" by what I'm eating because it's homemade, with organic ingredients that I took two whole seconds of undivided attention to select. And because, somehow, the sum of those variables seems to add up to something more than just good, healthy food. Somehow, it's satisfying on a much deeper level.

Like a hand that's fallen asleep that tingles as you wiggle your fingers and awaken it, I also remember the great, simple joy of eating. The unadulterated pleasure of eating that, mysteriously, I'd lost somewhere along the way while scarfing down microwaved junk with a plastic fork as I simultaneously took calls and answered emails and kept the corporate barracudas at bay before cramming my feet back into heels, still chewing my last frantic bite, and hustling down the hall to my next meeting.

There must be a job where work-life is healthier, more balanced, less consuming…and I'm pretty sure it's not in finance. So until I find it, I'll comb the usual websites, take on some freelance projects, and try to resist the riptide of anxiety that has highjacked me in the past. For the first time in my life, I'm going to really consider the next step, instead of continuing to repeat my career *samskarra* of allowing anxiety to propel me into yet another unfulfilling position, toxic environment, or terrible boss.

There's also the *Seva* Rotation to consider. Although I'd enrolled in the training as a life raft, teaching now seems like something I actually want to try. Yoga has helped me in so many ways...from pulling me out of heartbreak, to helping me survive my corporate existence, and now, as a tool to decrease my anxiety. My gratitude would be best expressed in passing it on to serve others. That the proceeds of the classes go to fund rescuing sweet little animals is even more reason to do it.

And just like that, I email Thea to accept a *Seva* Rotation and segue into the next chapter of my life.

Committing to teaching means I have to finish my assisting hours and submit my individual project in order to actually obtain my certificate. Under deadline and out of excuses, I face writing a paper about my final project. It's been over a year, but I'm finally making progress on lowering my anxiety. In fact, during my new home practices, I'd started to notice that I'm able to be more present and mentally still—sometimes even for a full 90 minutes. Practically an eternity! And during *savasana*, lying down on the mat, I can feel with greater awareness everything from the warm breeze blowing in the window, to the sounds of the intermittent traffic below, but I notice without trying to notice and without it distracting me.

Reaching this stillness is an achievement in and of itself. Surely, it warrants a medal, a pedestal, and a hearty rendition of the "Star-Spangled Banner." But the crowning achievement is that I've gotten to it on my own. In the solitude and challenge of my own practice, I've proven to myself that it's possible. The key to reaching this calm, focused state of stillness wasn't perfect prose or the expert guidance of a renowned teacher. It was the unsexy drudgery of small steps, the discipline of a slow pace, and wanting it badly enough to undergo the terrifying process of changing deeply ingrained patterns.

In freeing myself from those mental bonds, and with the benefit of space out-side Investorcap's walls, I also realize that it wasn't solely the industry that had held me prisoner all those years—it was also my own mind-set. I was the one who'd al-lowed myself to become utterly consumed by my job. I was the one who hadn't set strong enough boundaries around my time and energy. Investorcap hadn't sent an HR rep to follow me home and taunt me with to-do lists at four in the morning. In-vestorcap had never said I couldn't be more aware of what I was eating. Investorcap had never told me I couldn't take a vacation. Sure, Investorcap *had* piled on more work than one human could possibly do in this lifetime and denied me the infrastruc-ture and resources to actually do it, but I was the one who'd tried to do it anyway instead of telling them to go pee up a rain pipe. I was the one who'd risen to the bait—toward that ever-sexy Sirens' song of trying to do and have it all. That was me. I could see that now. And because it was me, I could also change it.

I feel, in some strange way, that I'm starting to become the person that I was always meant to be. For the first time, it feels like I'm in exactly the right place in my life, instead of fighting against every aspect of it. Yes, sometimes the transition is rocky. I'm switching from a highly structured, extraordinarily busy corporate life, and the driven personality I'd developed to live it, to a comparatively slow life, lived deliberately. That sort of thing is implicitly rocky. And, of course, I get sucked back into the murky depths of anxiety by various external events and internal patterns, such as trying to figure out my next job. (Either my yoga bubble's walls are too per-meable or I'm just too realistic to be in the "Zen Zone" 24/7.) But overall, I feel like I'm getting better at this life thing.

Not to get all yogic and New Age-y, but it feels as though I'm shedding a false skin that I wore for far too long and am emerging a truer, better, more authentic ver-sion of myself.

Okay, fine, maybe I'll get just a little yogic. But not New Age-y—that's where I draw the line.

Chapter Twenty-Four

A Yoga Guru: If Ever Wrong, Never in Doubt

I'm crawling through a yoga desert toward the unreachable mirage of actually *getting my certificate.* Oh wait, I'm only logging more assisting hours. It turns out that 40 hours of assisting—one class at a time—takes quite a while.

Utilizing the free time I now have, I sign up for every available assisting slot. I click into an assisting groove. I'm no longer nervous. I'm the mac daddy of assisting.

Thea approaches me after class one night. "Only 500-hour trainees are eligible to assist me at national conferences, but your skills are at that level if you're interested."

My heart swells. Travel with Thea to national conferences? The honor of it overwhelms me, but I try to play it cool. "Yeah! I mean, that'd be great."

I'm still floating on the accolade Thea's bestowed on me when I arrive to assist her next class a few days later.

In a shocking twist that nobody could've anticipated, Gloria and Summer, my two co-assistants, apparently not feeling bound by the concept of responsibility, don't show up. So I will now assist a packed class—45 students altogether—by my-self.

A student-assistant ratio of 45:1 doesn't bode well for me. My only consolation is my recent promotion to national assistant.

During the drop-in and breathwork, students kneel neatly on their mats, errone-ously making it seem that I may actually be able to handle this alone. Maybe I can impress Thea even more with some yoga Jedi moves I don't even know I have. On some level, I recognize that I'll probably be doomed shortly (I am only human after all...*one* human), but the ax hasn't fallen yet. A few moments later, Thea begins active practice and *whoosh*—it falls. At the same time, it becomes clear to me that at least one student is just as screwed as I am.

She's a frail, older woman. In her first downward-facing dog, her arms are already shaking, which means she lacks the overall strength and stamina to survive this advanced-level class. She's struggling mightily, and it's only going to go downhill from here as the class progresses. Thea's just beginning the warm-up.

I approach and ask if she's like to do restorative yoga instead—an option she gratefully accepts. I set her up in side-lying pose—a very basic pose consisting of...wait for it...*lying on your side.* As Thea taught us in the restorative workshop, the student is propped with blankets supporting the knees and another blanket under the shoulder on the floor.

No sooner do I finish than Thea appears like a genie. "The blanket goes under the side waist, not the shoulder."

I freeze under the glare of the correction. In light of my recent promotion to national assistant, my first instinct is the standard Tri Dosha robotic deference. But I'm sure I'm right about the shoulder because if there's one thing I know, it's that my anxiety drove me to study the manual until I knew it inside out and backward. See? There *is* a benefit to my anxiety. The only explanation is that she's revised it, which is fine, but I need to be kept up to date. "Wait, I'm confused. Has it changed since our training?"

"No. We've *always* done it that way." She's still smiling, but she makes it clear there's no two way about it and she's pissed I'd even ask.

She's so sure, I start to doubt myself. After all, as she told us in the training, she personally wrote the manuals and had the accompanying illustrations commissioned. I look around at the students, all parked in a low lunge. I'm not going to prolong their misery or compromise our professionalism by questioning her further. I have the manual, tucked like a security blanket, in my tote bag. I'll check it after the class and continue this with her then. "Okay," I say to Thea. I kneel beside the student. "Can you please sit up for a moment?" I ask. She does and I make the adjustment.

Thea walks away. The class and, therefore, my assisting duties resume. Grossly outnumbered, I'm the modern-day equivalent of the little Dutch boy with his finger in the dike, stemming an imminent flood of yoga disasters as I zoom around the huge studio making adjustments and fetching more props as they're requested. If I ever have a spare second to glance up at the front, I see Thea pointing to someone who's doing something wrong. Or at least, not to her liking. Who it is and what their crime is, however, I have no idea. There are 45 individuals—which comes to 180 limbs— flailing about, creating a veritable latticework that I can't see through. Plus, I'm desperately trying not to get nailed by any extremities as they lunge into the next *asana*. My assisting patrol takes on a strange sort of dance where I lunge and twirl out of danger.

As the practice rolls on, the air becomes hot and moist. I'm dying to step outside for a breath of crisp, fresh air but this is equally unacceptable on two counts: it could break the tenuous web of collective stillness the students are creating, and I'd risk annoying Thea. I can imagine her saying something along the lines of, "Sara, perhaps you need to look at the concepts of heat and sweat and your relationship to them," as she stares straight into my soul with a disapproving frown.

When I'm a student, I relish the heat, proud that my hard work contributed to it, sweating out my toxins, cleansing my pores, erasing whatever stress has lingered from the day with the effort I'm exerting on the mat. It feels like soul-deep purification, liberation even. Working deep into each pose, I revel in the heat, dive into it like a ring of fire, fearless, letting it transport me to a realm of post-exertion bliss.

I never realized, however, that from the teacher/assistant perspective, when you're not working in synchronicity with the rest of the room, the sweat-moistened heat just feels stifling. When I'm on the journey, it feels pivotal. When I'm helping to lead the journey, separate and detached from the student base, I feel like I should go home and do my own sweaty practice, except I'll be so tired from watching, assisting, and adjusting that I know I won't. This is no doubt akin to the difference between being a guest at a resort and being a resort employee. It's the same location, but two totally different experiences.

I swallow these thoughts and continue working. The class is already running impressively late—a fact I'm painfully aware of as I compulsively watch the clock and each nanosecond stretches into an eon. Thea appears unaware of time altogether.

I weave around students and wipe my sweaty forehead with my wrist. Being ever-vigilant as I analyze the alignment of every student and apply my arsenal of assists to them, is, in fact, *grueling*. Similar to when I used to be trapped in some brain-numbing meeting, I find myself staring out the window periodically just to escape, visually at least.

Is this what it'll be like to teach? If so, I think I'd rather stay a student.

Finally, finally…blessed *finally*, Thea ends the class, bringing everyone into *savasana,* corpse pose. In yet another shocking twist to this night, her lack of punctuality has turned what should've been a 90-minute class into an interminable two hours.

I exhale deeply, thankful it's over.

Thea perches on her block at the front. I zigzag around, wondering where to sit—next to her (we're a team?), behind her (in deference to her genius?), nowhere near her (I'm an island unto myself, removed from this yoga equation?). Striking a compromise, I finally settle on being off to the side. The students rest in *savasana*, cleansed and rejuvenated, relaxed and vibrant. Meanwhile, I'm charged up, nerves jangled, anxious and weary all at once. I try not to fidget. I don't want to disturb anyone.

Eventually, Thea gently guides the students back from repose into wakefulness. We chant three rounds of OM together, bow, and the students slowly wander out. I head toward the rejuvenation zone, also known as the locker room with sweet amenities.

I dig out the manual from the bottom of my tote, and flip through until I find side-lying pose. Sure enough, I see that the illustration shows the blanket under the shoulder. In case that leaves even a shadow of a doubt, the text below also clearly says the shoulder and nothing else. I roll it up and head toward the front desk, where Thea is giving her class count sheet to a kimono-clad attendant.

"Hey," I say, unrolling the manual and falling into step with her as she heads outside. "About side-lying pose, I just want to understand…because here's the illustration showing the shoulder. If it's changed, can you just let me know how we're doing it now?"

"It hasn't changed," she insists, really irritated now, but managing to keep a lid on it. She carefully examines the page I hold out to her. "Well Sara, you can't just go by the illustrations." Her tone is condescending. I wonder why *not* since she had an illustrator custom create them for her. But for the sake of cordiality, I keep that to myself. "You have to *read* the *written* directions," she continues, pointing to the text below.

In silence, heads bowed over the workbook, we read it together. Sure enough, the words haven't rearranged themselves in the past two minutes. It still says shoulder. "Well...we can't fit every single instruction in here," she argues, gesturing to a half-blank page with oodles of room.

I look at all the empty space dubiously. "Um...okay. But it doesn't say 'side waist' anywhere. Can you just...clarify?"

She reads it again, as though I'm lying—as though the words might really rearrange themselves this time. "Well...we didn't even really cover this pose in the training. We focused on others."

That alone is a problem—we should've thoroughly covered every pose in the manual. Otherwise, why include them at all? "But it's in your book and it was in your training," I protest, wondering why she won't just admit that she's wrong. I can intellectually respect anyone who admits they made a mistake or changed their mind—we're all only human after all—but I can neither respect nor understand Thea's compulsion to deny those human tendencies.

Concurrently, I wonder whatever happened to that whole thing about "being willing to be seen as human and humble, to show humility in your imperfection" that Thea had talked about at the last workshop. Hadn't she said that nobody can connect to ostensible perfection? Yet here she is, disregarding her own advice. I don't know what to do—battle it out with her? Call her out on this second level of inconsistency? Let the whole damnable thing go?

Somehow, in a move of sheer verbal wizardry that I will never fully comprehend, she neatly evades me by changing the topic to how the studio needs new props, and a moment later, she's gone.

As I drive home, I replay the entire interaction. Whether a blanket goes under the shoulder or the ribcage in any given pose is unimportant in the grand scheme of the cosmos. But the real conundrum was what our trivial battle represented.

Other issues aside, there's no doubt that Thea's an extraordinarily talented yoga teacher. She can look at a body and know its history, challenges, and possibilities. She creates sequences and leads them in such a way that provides an instrument for students to experience potentially life-changing transformations. Through the conduit of her training, I've questioned old patterns and worked hard to change them. That transformation alone was worthwhile. I'm thankful for it, as well as for her providing an indisputably thorough base for my future teaching.

But Thea is far from perfect. And it is perhaps her inability to admit that very obvious, very human fact that is her greatest deficiency. Maybe if she wasn't surrounded by yoga toadies (yoadies?), she might be better able to admit her flaws.

Although it's hardly fair to foist all the responsibility on the yoadies. Within the confines of the training, the only thing stronger than the smell of sweaty feet was the unfortunate stench of co-dependence. Some of the trainees seemed to have needed Thea in ways that Jessica and I simply didn't. They were the ones who'd arrived early to stake out spots nearest her, were frequently guilty of quoting her, and found any opportunity to fervently agree with or compliment her. This was done with a systematic thoroughness that could only be described as fanatical. The dynamic of hero worship was foreign to my nature. I could only assume that the yoadies derived some sort of validation through their very proximity to her, or maybe through receiving approval from her.

If I were to ever confront Thea on this point—not a tempting option if, in the language of financial services, past performance was any indication of future results—she'd probably find a way to once again turn it all back around on me. Just like the time she'd outed me for my anxiety when I suggested that exercise is good for the heart, or announced that "*Sara* really needs to eat," when I suggested that the class needed lunch breaks, or announced to everyone that I needed to examine my issues with chaos after I pointed out that the first community class was hopelessly chaotic. If I ever mustered the nerve to confront her about her own issues, I could imagine her telling me I needed to examine my relationship with authority or something. And for all I know, she might be right. I'd never claimed to know anything about subconscious psychological motivators and I was happily hell and gone from any sort of perfection.

But I did have eyes, ears, and a darn-near flawless memory. And, if I were to flip the script, I'd say that from my perspective, Thea was responsible for surrounding herself with servile flatterers who happily told her she was never wrong. She was equally responsible for believing it. Sure, the yoadies were responsible for worshipping a highly imperfect human as some sort of guru, but she was responsible for receiving or fostering it. One party can't be blamed for co-dependence. It takes a certain kind of person on both sides of the dynamic for it to exist at all.

A healthier paradigm might be for leaders to solicit questions, discussion, and continuous evaluation, and to be open to all responses. If my experience in the corporate world is a blueprint at all, leaders surrounding themselves with yes-men is never the way forward. But in order for this to work, the guru/leader has to be receptive to questions, discussions, and continuous evaluation. And, the problem as I see it, is that this one is not.

Chapter Twenty-Five

The Student Becomes the Teacher

Impatiently, I wait for Thea to send my certification, wondering if maybe she's still mad about our last confrontation, or hasn't had time to read the paper I wrote about my individual project, or if, perhaps, she didn't consider it good enough. Regardless, I need to know. I email to inquire about its status and she responds with it as an attachment. There's no message. Anticlimactically, it's just a plain Microsoft Word document with my name and 200-hour designation. Jessica receives her certificate as well—with the name Kate on it.

Ah, yoga people. Some things will never change.

I can't believe it: my training is finally complete. Done. Over. *Finito.* Two years from the time I applied, I'm finally a certified yoga teacher. I twirl around the apartment. I feel like doing cartwheels down the street. *I'm a certified yoga teacher!* If I had any talent, I'd sing.

In preparation for teaching my first *Seva* class—my very first class *ever!*—I sit down at the computer to design my sequence. I'm still of corporate heritage; all work is done on computers, even yoga sequences. And it had better be good because I have to log it in an online repository, along with my thoughts on teaching, for Thea and her 500-hour students to review. Additionally, the 500-hour students will be dropping in for surprise check-ups. I have 15 days to prepare.

I wonder what my students will be like, what they'll think about me. I coach myself to show strong leadership and boundaries, but also be kind and approachable. I must be firm in my instruction, but also forgiving, popular, but not obviously interested in being so, inspired and inspiring. I want to be the teacher who illuminates the path, the one they recall as life-changing years later, but humble and open about my many imperfections.

My classes themselves will be composed of architecturally brilliant sequences. Since it's a mixed-level class, it needs to be both accessible to beginners and challenging for the advanced. I want the experience to be a sparkling lagoon in the jungle of a Sunday. Students will emerge refreshed and rejuvenated.

The class is only an hour and a half, but hey, I figure that's do-able, right? Uh...*right?*

I stare at the blank screen; the blank screen stares back. I try to think of poses, but I can't seem to remember anything other than sun salutations and I'm so sick of them, I just might puke if I have to do one more. Yes, I know that's super yogic of me, but I can't help thinking of them as the yoga equivalent of carnations or iceberg lettuce. Filler.

Half an hour passes. The screen is still blank. I go to the *Yoga Journal* website and browse their pose library.

I decide this is ridiculous. I should design it where it will be practiced. I roll out my mat, stack every handout and workbook from the training beside me, and prepare to spawn greatness.

"Introductions, welcome, ask for injuries," I write. God, it's good to have words on the page.

I start to sketch out a sequence, practicing each pose and transition as I go. The class needs to be 90 minutes in length—which seems to be an ocean-sized void to fill—but I spend so much time trying and then redoing, that I have no idea how long my sequence-in-progress actually is.

I practice it on myself the next day and get it down to 90 minutes exactly. But I am only one person. Will it take a class of 20-plus people longer because somehow groups always take longer despite the fact that groups are made up of individuals? Not to mention the additional incalculable delays of adjustments. How to account for those?

The next day, I ask my sister Hanna, a yoga novice, if she'll be my guinea pig. Yoga novice might be a bit of an exaggeration—she's only done yoga once before and that was when I dragged her to a class promising it would change her life. It hadn't, so she stopped. Given this, it's not surprising that the sequence looks com-pletely different—and much harder—on her.

"Dude. You killed my hamstrings," she says, hobbling out of my apartment.

Wimp, the older sister in me thinks. The newly budding yoga teacher in me ar-gues that since this is a mixed-level class, it's likely I'll have some yoga newbies and should probably adjust accordingly.

"I'm glad we got to hang out! Good bonding time!" I call down the stairs after her. There's no response.

I email Hazel and Jessica and ask if I can practice it on them. Experienced prac-titioners, the sequence now looks easy. Which probably means that it falls squarely in the middle ground. I hope that works.

I'm so nervous on the actual day of teaching my first class that I can barely eat. It's job-interview nerves, first-day-at-work nerves, and presentation-to-a-group nerves all rolled into one. The studio is only 20 minutes away, but I insist on leaving an hour early in case there is traffic and to allow time to look for parking. Nunnally reminds me that it's Sunday evening and there won't be any traffic, but I insist, irri-tated that he's not taking every precautionary measure to ensure a timely arrival. Doesn't he understand *anything*?

Of course, there's no traffic and I find a huge parking space directly in front of the studio, so we're quite early. Nunnally, who's coming to his second-ever class to support me, wisely doesn't gloat.

We sit outside—only a geek would arrive this early, the last class hasn't even ended yet and there are no students in the waiting area—and I compulsively read over my sequence. This is a time-honored study practice I developed in college: read the study material over and over and over. Read it again. When you finally feel like you'll vomit if you have to read it one more freaking time, then you know you're finally ready. Overpreparedness has always been my mantra. "Inhale and sweep your arms slowly overhead…(wait one beat)…exhale and draw them to your heart…(wait one beat)….” Argh! No more!

I wage an internal battle, trying to make myself read it *just one more time* while my brain flatly refuses, until it's finally time to go in. Then it's my body's turn to revolt: My feet don't want to walk where I'm telling them. They're refusing to carry me into the class. I stand frozen on the sidewalk. Panic surges. I'm terrified to go in. I might throw up.

Note to self: address crippling anxiety. Finally, I force myself through the front door, swearing I'll never do this again. I introduce myself to the volunteer at the front desk checking people in.

Nunnally goes ahead to set up his mat and props next to our friend Brian and my sister Annie, who's driven an hour to come support me. Hanna's hamstrings still haven't recovered. I hope Annie avoids the same fate.

I peek into the classroom. Everyone is seated or reclining on their mats, waiting for the teacher to call the class to attention. I have another sudden, panic-fueled desire to pivot on my heel and run as fast as I can, far away.

My anxiety intensifies to previously unknown levels. I remind myself that these people paid to take this class. I think of the rescued animals who will benefit from the proceeds. I roll my shoulders back, lift my chin, and go in.

There are only four people besides Nunnally, Annie, and Brian. From the back, it appears to be an accurate representation of the Back Bay beauties in full logo-ed splendor, highlights and lowlights perfectly streaking through their impeccable, bouncy ponytails. This is Boston after all. A wave of relief that everyone is clean and well kept sweeps over me. It's a stark contrast to the teacher training.

Unfortunately, I've been assigned a huge room that feels loft-like. The eight of us swim untethered in this over-large space. It reminds me of an empty restaurant. You walk in, see there's nobody else there, and quickly back out because surely the food can't be good—and even if it is, the waiter will hover over you, giving you his undivided attention, making you feel scrutinized, and thus ruining your meal.

I walk up to the front, legs shaking. I turn and face my students. The door opens and my stomach lurches as Jaznae strolls in. *Of course.* Perhaps more surprisingly, Brinley is in the front row. I'm already a terrified, shaky mess. But now, if I blow it, two people will actually *know.* They might also report it back to Thea.

My fears of public speaking and being watched surge forward. I try to push them back. I tell myself that being watched and speaking to groups are requirements of teaching, but this only leads me to the inescapable fact that I'm precisely the antithesis of who should be a teacher.

Anxiety's hallmarks kick in: I try to swallow, but my mouth has gone dry. There's a lump in my throat. I'm suddenly irritated and hot. I wish someone else were standing at the front, ready to be the teacher. I wish I were only walking *past* the front to get an extra block or something, but there is no one else up here. Just me. *Alone.*

I see Nunnally smiling encouragingly and mouthing, "I love you!" But his presence, meant to comfort me, actually makes my anxiety spike even more. And suddenly Brian's being there is kind of scary too since he has actually done yoga before. What if I don't measure up? Annie, at least, is a source of undiluted support. I could run over a puppy and Annie would find a way to be supportive. "Well…the puppy shouldn't have been in the street! You're a great driver!"

As I've been doing for the past year for my individual project, I reel my brain in and refocus on my breathwork. I get a blanket and blocks to stall for time. I keep doing calming breathwork and it actually starts to work…a little. I look at my 12 pages of notes and, voice shaking, ask if anyone's new or working with injuries. I sound like a fool, an imposter. I sound like I'm only pretending to be the teacher—which is, perhaps, fitting, given that I *feel* like I'm only pretending to be the teacher.

Jaznae raises her hand. Reluctantly, I make my way over. "Hello, Sara," she says regally. "I have a summer cold and I've been working way too hard lately… really overextending myself energetically. I'm going to college to get a degree in accounting."

I have a PTSD-fueled flashback to the immersion when Jaznae had claimed that higher education was a tool of the white man to oppress minorities. Or some such. I try to ignore that and focus on what she's saying.

"So…I may just do my own restorative practice tonight," she finishes.

I briefly wonder why she chose to come to an active, vigorous *vinyasa* class—and not just any *vinyasa* class, my debut class—if she wanted to do her own thing. Then I decide I have more important things to worry about. "Sounds good," I say, moving away.

She nods imperially, then slowly, dramatically, reclines down on her mat.

I head resignedly back to the teacher spot. "Okay," I say when I get there, "let's get started in *virasana*, hero's pose." I kneel on my mat and sit back on the blocks to demonstrate. I look around and Brinley's way ahead of me, eyes closed, doing dramatic *ujjiy* breathing that can probably be heard from Las Vegas. Ignoring her, I instruct the class to close their eyes. Once they aren't looking at me, I relax a bit. *A tiny bit.*

I walk them through the drop-in, the internally stilling process focusing on the breath, and *bandhas*, a series of muscular engagements to create energetic locks. I start with *mula bandha*, the root lock. I once was in a class where the teacher told us to engage our *mula bandhas* and as we did, to visualize them as beautiful pink lotus flowers. With each breath, she guided us to feel our lotus flower *mula bandhas* blossom open and closed.

Ah, that lotus analogy was lovely. It was magical. I'd immediately felt more yogic just hearing those poetic words.

If only I had known what the hell she was talking about, or where this lotus flower was supposed to be lodged, I could've practically reached enlightenment by the end of that class. But she didn't explain. So I had spent the class distracted by thoughts of where my lotus was and left in about the same state as when I walked in, except utterly confused.

So, for curious, detail-oriented students like me, I now decide to thoroughly explain *mula bandha*. "For those who may not know, the *bandhas* are a series of muscular and energetic locks throughout the body. *Mula bandha*, the root lock, consists of the engaging the pelvic floor muscles." It then occurs to me that not everyone knows these muscles. I continue, "For those who aren't sure what those are, they're the same muscles you'd use to do Kegel exercises." *Nice, DiVello, the men in the room—and maybe some of the women—might not know what Kegels are either.* I clarify further, "And in case anyone still doesn't know what I'm talking about, try a sequential engagement of the uro-genital and anal sphincter muscles. Then find the midway point between them and lift."

At the mention of "anal sphincter," Nunnally and Brian audibly choke back laughter, emitting poorly obstructed snarfing sounds as they do. *Boys.* I pointedly ignore them.

As we sit in v*irasana*, hero's pose, my fingertips graze my heels. Skin meets skin and I smile. I can't believe I'm working—albeit unpaid—and I get to be barefoot!

I think of my first class and how my feet bore the imprints from wearing high heels all day. Now I am free—literally and podiatrically—of the corporate world. Free!

I instruct everyone to deepen their *ujjiy* breath, and remember my very first class in the sweaty gym basement when I'd first tried and ended up coughing instead. Now I breathe deep, resonant breaths, soothing my nervous system with the familiar and calming rhythm. I watch the simplicity of physical stillness and focused breathing work their magic on those before me. I feel the same shift within myself.

Faces soften, foreheads unwrinkle, and jaws unclench. *Look, I'm helping people! I totally get this! I love this!* Encouraged, I ask everyone to create an intention for their practice. And as everyone finds their causes, I find my own: to stay calm and grounded through this first foray into teaching.

Then I remember that I have to lead the OM. In front of this sparsely attended class. *Please do not hang me out to dry—my voice empty and alone.* I peek and see the Beauties perching prettily on their mats, looking impeccable, ponytails perky.

"Adding sound to your intention, let's open our practice with a communal OM. Inhaling…" I inhale loudly to let them know the time is coming—hope vainly that someone will start the chorus for me, but of course nobody does—and valiantly let 'er rip. "OOOOOOOOOOOOOOOOOMMMMMMMMMMM…." I wait for the class to join me, but mine remains the only voice in the room. Here it is: my greatest embarrassment is happening. It's not unlike that infamous dream of being caught naked in public. I've never had that dream, but at this moment, I *feel* naked. My voice is utterly exposed, without covering or support from anyone else. It sounds sad and solitary in this too-big room, echoing by itself. My face gets hot. My voice cracks. Why the hell isn't Nunnally helping? What about Annie and Brian?

Abruptly, I wrap it up. But I'm still shaken. I want to cry. Instead, I take two shaky breaths and remember my goal—to give teaching a try, share the benefits I've experienced in my practice, and raise money for animal rescue. I ground myself and begin.

But as I transition to active practice, things start to really go awry. The class had been incorrectly listed as power yoga on the schedule, which at first I hoped wouldn't be a big deal. I now see, however, these students expect to zoom along mindlessly, aerobically working up a sweat. I get through the first sun salutation and they rev into competitive turbo-gear. They ignore my slow and deliberate directions. They are on autopilot, grinding through their usual practice. It's like watching a movie in fast-forward. I'm flustered, completely out of control, and mortified in front of Brinley and Jaznae.

The students lack the rudimentary body awareness needed to execute each pose safely. As I teach each pose, they toss out some bastardized version of it, but have no eye or interest in refining alignment or doing the work of yoga. Instead, they sacrifice these basic pillars in an effort to contort themselves into advanced positions beyond what I'm teaching…and their true ability levels.

As a first-time teacher, I'm not sure what to do about this. I stare, feeling helpless. These students have a lot of work ahead—work they apparently have no interest

271

in attempting. Kicking into desperation mode, I attempt the yoga equivalent of herding cats. And am predictably unsuccessful. This is a disaster.

In a last-ditch effort, I dare to disregard Thea's advice on not giving assists in the beginning stages of one's teaching career. Maybe I can turn this around, one student at a time.

As I attempt the impossible, teaching *and* assisting my first class, I suddenly realize why Thea advised against it. The challenge of assisting—scanning a roomful of bodies and trying to determine which assist should be given at which time to which student within the span of one pose—in addition to leading the class, guiding the sequence, and making sure we stay on time, is a little intense.

And by "a little intense," I mean, of course, "completely out of the freaking question."

A few times I adjust a Back Bay beauty and haven't moved two steps away before I see her revert to her original posture. I wonder if I'm to blame—*was my assist inaccurate? Can she see I have no clue what I'm doing? Or is it her? Is some underlying, deep-seated issue at work?*

Halfway into the class, Jaznae waves wildly. Trying not to lose my train of thought, I slowly work my way along the entire length of the room toward her. "May I have an extra blanket? My body needs to come into restorative," Jaznae intones when I'm still four people away. I assume this PYA (Public Yoga Announcement) is for the benefit of everyone around her.

I glance at the stack of blankets directly beside her. Still trying to stay focused on my verbal cues for the rest of the students, I retrieve one for her.

"An extra block as well?" she continues, eyes closed theatrically.

Gritting my teeth, I fetch it for her.

"Thank you," she says. Her tone says, "At last, the queen has been served."

"And now, stepping slowly back to downward-facing dog," I say to the class as I bring them into the next pose and return to my mission of focusing on an individual level. A prime opportunity is directly in front of me. I see that, at almost six feet tall, this Back Bay beauty's compressed herself into a downward-facing dog suitable for a much smaller person. It's like watching Shaquille O'Neal trying to be in Danny DeVito's down dog.

Wait—that sounds kind of weird, but you know what I mean. Instead of seeing her gracefully stretched out, her compressed stance is creating muscle constriction in her neck and shoulders, preventing her from finding overall ease, length in the neck, and breadth in the shoulders. Basically, she's squashing herself. Inevitably, her breath is nonexistent because her chest is compacted and her body is tensing in discomfort. "I'm going to make a gentle shoulder adjustment now," I say, just like Thea taught us so as not to startle the inverted student.

She snaps her head up. "No." The word is rigid and unyielding—exactly like her pose.

Startled, I take half a step back. I've never seen anyone refuse an assist in *any* class I've ever attended in over a decade of doing yoga. Thinking she must not have understood my intent, I quietly explain the ramifications of her compression on her neck and shoulders, and the domino effects through the rest of her pose.

"I *said* I'm *not* changing!" She yells loudly. "I'm fine just like this!"

I freeze. On mats around us, heads whip up and people stare. In the silence of the practice, she might as well have screamed into a bullhorn.

The stubborn part of myself, the fighter, the corporate me, wants to take her on. I want to show her the light because I can clearly see that she's wrong. I want to force her to accept my help and change to a healthier pose. The yoga part of me recognizes that she's got her own stuff going on and I can't interfere with whatever that is. The self-conscious part of me just wants this interaction to end because I'm freaking *mortified*. These internal sides wage war for a long moment, then I surrender and walk away.

As the class grinds on, it occurs to me that maybe I'm the one who didn't get the memo: this is listed as *power yoga*. The Beauties are here for a *workout*.

Yet in spite of this obvious fact, I blame their lackluster practice on myself because surely if I were a better teacher, a stronger teacher, a more compassionate teacher, I'd be able to bridge this gap for them. I'd hurl myself across the crevasse like one of those bridges made of rope in a movie jungle scene, and let my students cross safely toward more-evolved versions of themselves.

Instead, I have everyone in a hamstring-lengthening forward bend and Shaquille Devito whips up into a headstand. When it's time for an inversion and I teach shoulder stand, she loudly demands, "Can't we do headstand instead? We *always* do headstand."

I grit my teeth. It's clearly become a power struggle. Even her complaining question feels aggressive. "If that's what your body is asking for," I reply, tiptoeing around a quicksand bog of her issues, desperately trying not to get sucked in.

I need to reestablish order. The rest of the class needs to know Shaquille Devito is an aberration. I walk to the front. "Yoga is a place to find balance between effort and surrender," I begin. "Take this time to listen to what your body is asking you for, turning away from ego." Clearly I'm not all yogic myself; I can't help throwing in that last part. I glance at Brinley and Jaznae, wondering if this will go in their reports to Thea.

I consider it a minor victory when all the other students opt to do the shoulder stand I was teaching in the first place. Okay, so if the yoga didn't reach Shaquille Devito this time, at least it brushed the other students with a tinge of awareness. I may not have succeeded in my desire to illuminate the yogic path, but at least I got some people to slow down and tune in to what felt right instead of what they "always" did. That at least was something.

But it isn't everything. As we head toward the end of the class, Shaquille Devito simply stands, hands on hips, and refuses to do any pose at all. Glancing nervously at her, I keep going, but I'm thoroughly rattled.

"And now moving back to dogward-facing down." In my state of angst, I flub arguably one of the most well-known poses. "Uh...I mean downward-facing dog," I correct. Two girls laugh—and not in the much-joked about "laughing *with* you" way. No, this is actually *at* me. Unkindly. I spiral into acute self-consciousness.

Finally, I bring the class into *savasana*. As the students rest, I focus on doing calming breathwork. Inhale...extend the exhale. Inhale...extend the exhale. Inhale...try not to cry. Or worry about what Brinley might tell Thea. Inhale...ignore Jaznae.

Determined to end the class on time at least, I bring the students back up to a seated position. *Everyone* patently refuses to chant OM. So once again, I OM alone. Hearing my own voice unaccompanied and unaided makes me feel like an even bigger loser.

I suddenly miss the training community—in spite of their quirks, flaws, and sometimes questionable hygiene. At least they "get" the work of yoga. They want it. They're *open* to it. I now realize these qualities are important to me.

Jaznae rolls up her mat and heads for the door without a word. I raise my chin—proud that at least I didn't let her get to me. On her way out, Brinley pauses near me, and I remember how nice she was to reach out to me when I got kicked out of my group. Maybe she's not here to spy. Maybe she's here to support me. "Thanks for coming," I tell her. "If there's anything I can work on, please let me know." Foolishly, I'm eager for her approval, for any tiny scrap of acknowledgment for successfully completing my first class.

She looks at me without expression. "The only thing I can say is: don't worry—you'll get better." *Zing!* With one foul, fell swoop, she whooshed in and smashed any budding confidence.

Shaquille Devito glares at me one final time, grabs her mat, and stomps out. I'm shaken by her anger. I resist—barely—the desire to curl into fetal pose and go to my happy place.

"That was great!" Annie says, standing on her tip toes for a hug. I'm a head taller.

"No, not really," I say, hunching down and hugging, but also watching over her shoulder as the door slams behind Shaquille Devito.

"Yes, really!" Annie assures me, supportive to the end.

Annie leaves to start her long drive home. Brian gives me a thumbs-up and heads out as well. Nunnally goes to take a shower. I pad around the empty studio, putting away props that people left out. It reminds me of naptime the summer I worked as a nanny—the house steeped in quiet, picking up after the kids while they slept upstairs. When the studio is tidy, I meet Nunnally in the lobby. "Bye! Thank you!" I call cheerily to the front desk volunteer.

"Why didn't you guys OM? with me?" I demand as soon as we're in the privacy of the car, all trace of cheer gone.

"What? I was supposed to OM with you? Nobody else did. I thought it was something the teacher did by herself."

"No. It's supposed to be everyone, but they totally hung me out to dry. Why do you think you were there anyway? Oh God—and I sounded so awful!" I bite back a sob.

"You sounded good," Nunnally assures me.

"Whatever," I say, escaping into that one word conversation-ender. "In the future, don't make me OM alone."

"Don't worry, there won't be an OM alone two," Nunnally jokes.

Later, safely ensconced in the comfort of my couch with a hearty glass of red wine, the dark cloud of the class still hangs over me, but the interaction with Shaquille Devito was the most upsetting. It wasn't just the level of her anger, which seemed disproportionate for the horrifying crime of offering her an adjustment. And it wasn't the bizarre incongruity of her trying to reduce her attention-attracting height while at the same time choosing attention-seeking, often unsafe versions of the poses I was teaching. It wasn't even the fact that she had paradoxically rejected my teaching and done her own thing when she was, in fact, choosing to attend my class instead of practicing at home by herself.

What really got to me was how utterly closed she was to the idea of trying something different, of *change*. It was her sheer immovability, her words: *I'm* not *changing.*

Given my own status as a towering giantess, of course I understood wanting to be smaller. I knew all too well what it was like to wish that you were average height, to have spent your whole life looming over most of the dating pool. In the same way that I hunched my way through my teen years desperately wanting to be tiny and delicate, she was hunching her way through her practice. That much, I got. I could even understand wanting attention, although I usually preferred a seat in the wings instead of the spotlight.

But what I absolutely could not get was her refusal to consider change when the effects of her compression, and the compression itself, were brought to her attention.

Then again, I consider all the people in the I'm-not-changing boat. A parade of my bosses and fellow yoga trainees flashes through my mind. I could probably think of innumerable others, even some friends and family.

The question of why is simple: Because ultimately it's easier, and far more comfortable, to continue doing what you've always done, instead of asking the harder questions that can lead to the scarier choices, like what might be possible if you let go of what you've always done?

Isn't that what had kept me, trapped but safe, in financial services for so long?

Chapter Twenty-Six
The Quest to Fit In…at Any Cost

Big news: one of the coolest purveyors of yoga fashion has opened a store in Boston. I troll the downtown location, looking at the broad array of colors and patterns and, feeling like a five-year old in a toy store, grab everything I can get my overeager mitts on and head to the dressing room.

There, something bizarre happens. My size is not fitting me. At all. And not just off by an inch. I mean, really not fitting. As in, I can't get the shirts over my head or the pants up over my hips. I go up a size, but no visible progress is made.

I insist to myself that they *will* fit and cram myself into a beautiful raspberry top. I promptly get stuck—arms flailing like a disembodied octopus. Ultimate humiliation, I have to call for help and have some poor salesgirl wrestle me out of it.

To her credit—and I do give her credit, as I am not sure I could have refrained from laughing—she's kind and dignified. She tries to help tug me out of it.

No dice.

She tries to dig her fingers in between my flesh and the top.

She can't.

She stands on a bench and tries to pull it over my head.

Not happening.

Finally, heroically, she bends her knees, braces her legs, and pulls with all her might, emitting a mighty grunt as she does so.

Still nothing.

There is one brief second where she indicates defeat—she can't get me out of it—and true panic sets in. *Will I be stuck in this forever? Will they be forced to call for scissors and cut me out of it? Oh God…will I have to pay for it if they do?* Eventually, however, she manages the impossible (thankfully, without a tub of Vaseline) and I am freed.

I briefly debate hightailing it out of there, anxious to escape the humiliation of being pried out of a piece of clothing in a public setting, but my dogged determination wins out. I will not let this deter me in my mission. Deciding it's just this *particular* top, I go back and grab a sample of every style they offer, several sizes larger than my usual. But I find that if something fits in the chest, it hangs like a tent around my waist. If it fits in the waist, there's no way I can get it up over my breasts.

If I actually manage to wrangle myself into a pair of pants, they're so long they look like footed PJs. Feeling suddenly like the proverbial square block in a round hole (and really, who's the hole in this scenario?), and getting sweatier and more frustrated by the nanosecond, I set my jaw and go to the stubborn place. *Oh, I will find something that fits. Today. Just freaking watch me. I. Will. Make. This. Happen.*

Objectively, I recognize this strikes a deep-seated chord within me. I've spent my entire life wanting to be something I wasn't. My sister Hanna has always had a ridiculously perfect, thick, glorious mass of French curls adorning her perfect little head. I've wanted those curls ever since she grew that head of hair, when she was about two and I was seven, jealously looking on with my fine, thin sprig of a ponytail.

I have also always wanted to be tiny and delicate, a mere feminine wisp of a thing, like Annie. When you are Annie's height, you can shift your eyes flirtatiously up to look at men and seem cute and graceful while doing so. When you are Annie's height, men (and some women for that matter) open doors for you and offer to help you carry your bags/suitcase/groceries/purse/whatever you might be carrying.

When you're my height, you stare straight across at most men, and down at a fair share as well. When you're my height, you're expected to hold doors and help people Annie's height carry their stuff. When you're my height, it's hard to feel feminine and delicate, let alone find good clothes that fit right.

So starting from about the age of 11, when I was already a concerning 5'7" and had started to develop outward as well, I started to include specifications in my nightly prayers regarding my continued growth. They went something along the lines of: "Thank you, God, for all the things you give me." And here I would pause for a moment in gratitude, because to rush directly into asking for what I wanted seemed rude. And I'd wonder how long I should politely wait before desperately adding my requests: "Please God, don't let me grow any taller and don't let my boobs get any bigger than an A-cup. *Please*, God, *please*."

It had seemed greedy to ask for perfect French curls too, so I'd stuck to the top-priority items, figuring once I stopped growing, I could get a perm. (A separate disaster.)

By age 13, I'd passed 5'8", which made me taller than all the girls I knew, and my feet were already a size eight. There I was, a giantess in a land of delicate nymphs, anchored by giant clodhoppers. Of course, I was also taller than all the boys, which was way worse. *Hello? How would anyone ever ask me out at this horrific, towering height and with these ungraceful, ginormous feet?* My boobs, too, kept expanding despite my best smoosh and hide. I refused to move on from a training bra until I was literally spilling over and below and out of it. I became a professional sloucher as I reached my final destination at well over 5'9" and a generous C-cup.

So Annie got the height, politely stopping her growing at a petite 5'4", and Hanna got the curls, the maintenance of which she had the audacity to complain about, and I got neither. And to top it off, to really rub salt in my self-conscious wounds, I also didn't get the boobs I'd wanted. And when you're at the peak of female self-conscious, gawky awkwardness, it seemed life just wasn't fair. I continued with my slouch-and-hide campaign well into college.

Now, to be fair, this impression of mine wasn't just the product of acute self-consciousness and overexaggeration. In fact, if it had not been created, it had certainly been reinforced, by the world around me. For instance, I once rented a car to drive to Philly to visit my family because my 14-year old Blazer couldn't make such a long journey. So I found an online deal—some steep discount for the "ultra econo-model." The online picture had shown a powder blue, two-door hatchback. However, when I arrived in person to pick it up, the dubious, diminutive Latino man behind the counter had shaken his head and said, "Oh, no. Oh no, no, *no*! You need upgrade. You very *beeg* girl. You no gonna fit in leetle car. I get you beeg car for free."

I started to protest at my gargantuan "beeg" size, "No, really, I want the cute, little car. Please! Give me the little one!" (Note to self: do not ever scream, "Give me the little one!" in public. Or ever.) But he waved me off. "No, no. No problema, mami. Eet's okay. You way too beeg. I take care of." And with that, I was placed, free of charge, into a four-door family car that was apparently large enough to accommodate even my mammoth stature.

Despite this particularly scarring incident, somewhere toward my mid-twenties, I started to get more comfortable. Befriending a few fellow tall girls certainly helped, as did my Aunt Pat once looking me straight in the eye and stating with absolute certainty, "A woman cannot be considered beautiful under 5'9"."

Aunt Pat knew these things. She wore Chanel perfume. The concept of meeting the beauty requirement was new; I loved it.

But faced with a situation such as my current one—stuck in a dressing room with my body refusing to conform to the ideals that I want it to—brings that self-consciousness roaring back to the surface. It only intensifies my desire to find something that *does* fit, come hell or high water.

I spend over two hours trying on clothes, determined that something will fit me, and getting progressively more frustrated, sweaty, and hysterical in the process. Yoga breathing and anti-anxiety measures apparently decided to wait outside for me.

In the end, I cram myself into a too-small top, ignoring that it creates the kind of cleavage you just don't see in a regular, run-of-the-mill yoga class and a pair of pants that I'll have to hem by six inches, and run out of the store, shaken but victorious.

Proud of my hard-won trophies, I wear the shirt to class the next day. I'm just outside the heavy, sliding door, about to head in, when I see a former teacher named Veronica leaving for the night.

She waves. "Sara! Hi!"

All I really want to do is go claim a wall spot, get my props, and get settled, but feeling guilty for no longer going to her classes, I walk over to give her a hug. "Hey! How are you?"

"Wow. You have fantastic tits!" she says, staring.

Surely, I've misheard her. Obviously, the dynamics of the hallway have warped her words. I must look confused because she leans in closer and says louder, so that I can't possibly misunderstand, "Seriously, you have the most fantastic tits!"

I flush and step back, mortified. "Um…thank you?"

She nods. "So how was your weekend?"

Eventually, I escape to the class, now acutely self-conscious about my prominently squashed cleavage. Every few minutes, the word "tits" replays in my brain like mental Tourette's. Even Thea's boss-like tone can't drown this out. "And from *parsvokonasana*, slowly raising the right arm…" *TITS!* "…and stepping back to downward facing dog…" *TITS!* "…and now, lunge gently forward, keeping the knee over the ankle…" *TITS!*

These battles—with both shirt and brain—distract me utterly and entirely from the yoga. I guess I'm just not meant to fit into this yoga brand. And I guess I'm not yogic enough to stay present. *Double whammy.*

I think back to the corporate-wear—button-down shirts that never fit right, constricting suits, pinchy high heels—and how I never felt like I belonged in the clothes or the conference rooms. Now I'm in my new world, but the "uniform" doesn't fit any better.

Perhaps it is my karma to not fit in anywhere.

Chapter Twenty-Seven

The Zen Within and the Zen for Them

I'm almost as nervous and twice as filled with dread when I go back the following week to teach my second *Seva* class because now I know what to expect. Indeed, it *is* as bad as I remember. Worse perhaps because I'm utterly alone, Nunnally is stuck working. Brian and Annie had prior obligations—or at least claimed they did.

Only three girls show up this time, and only one is a return customer. Another snaps her gum loudly. I briefly consider demanding that she spit it in my hand like my first teacher did, but shudder and decide not to. Everything from the room to the energy is grim and difficult, the antithesis of yoga. Everyone churns mechanically, swiftly, efficiently through their practice. No one takes time to explore—or even to simply feel—the poses.

The fighter in me wants to duke this out. *I* will *bring you around*, I think, setting my jaw and feeling irrationally annoyed by my floppy, apathetic students. The tired-of-fighting-and-trying-to-be-yogic part of me wonders if it wouldn't be better to give up now, leaving this class to a more aerobically minded instructor who doesn't care about things like mindfulness and refining alignment.

The fighter wins out, but desperate yoga measures must be taken. So, on the third class I decide to break Thea's rule of a silent practice. In the Tri Dosha world, this is, indeed, a desperate measure. It was practically a cardinal sin, way worse than carnivory or drinking coffee.

Nonetheless, I bring a folk and easy listening playlist that took me all day to create and choreograph my sequence to. I feel pretty darn proud of this minor accomplishment...until one girl stops practicing altogether, sits up on her mat, and starts singing along.

Note to self: only use music without *lyrics.*

Every week I swim upstream. I bring my A-game. The few students who show up act like they're doing me a huge favor just by dragging their bored, toned asses there. You'd think yoga was court-ordered community service. It's hard to keep pumping energy into the void. But I'm determined to stick it out even though what I really want to do is throw in the towel, say I was just kidding about this whole teaching thing, and go running straight back to my comfort zone at a desk.

Stubbornly, I decide to stick to my principles or go down with the ship. I do, however, crank up the difficulty level to a point that even I could barely manage on my best days. I'm determined to make them deepen their breath, work harder, and respect the work of this class at any cost.

In spite of past performance, I know this class can get to the Zen yoga place. After all, if it's possible for an obsessive-compulsive, anxiety-ridden worrier of freakish proportions such as myself to shift to meditative mental silence for the length of a class, it's possible for anyone. The path is there, comprised of practical efforts. And I can help them reach it. I just have to stay the course.

A few weeks later, I'm straightening up after yet another grim, sparsely attended class when the studio manager comes in. She's training a new front desk girl tonight, otherwise she's long gone by the time I arrive. "How's it going?" she asks, grabbing the Swiffer.

"Really well, I think," I lie.

"You're doing great. This is a tough timeslot, being so late. It really makes eating dinner at the *ayurvedic* time challenging." I nod as though I know what she's talking about and it's really challenging for me too, and she continues, "So we have an open teaching slot and I thought you might be a good fit."

My heart soars. "Wow! Really? I mean, thank you so much! I'm thrilled! Yes, I'd love it." Suddenly I don't mind the apathetic students. The studio values me and my work. Hooray!

She raises one hand and gives a gentle, little laugh. "Don't get too excited. It's an eight pm class on Mondays, so it's about the same as this one…you know, not the most popular timeslot…." She says this to temper my enthusiasm with reality. Teachers get paid on a per-student commission here. "But it's a good starting point for a new teacher."

I nod, still thrilled. "Absolutely," I agree. I'm the equivalent of a recent college grad. I've only just started an internship here. Of course I'm not going to get the prime time slots right away. It's a huge honor to be offered a real class and it's exciting that I got it on my own. It will be wholly and utterly mine—unlike the *Seva* class, I won't have to record my sequences and thoughts on teaching for Thea's review and approval (even though she'd never actually commented or sent me feedback, it was still stressful knowing she was electronically watching). I won't have to worry about surprise visits from the 500-hour trainees. I'll be officially venturing out on my own—without the support or the burden of Thea or the Tri Dosha community. It's equally terrifying and exhilarating.

I roll down all the windows on the drive home. It's a perfect, still-hot summer night, the kind that makes you crave barbeque, cornbread, and sweet tea. The warm air blows across my bare arms as I cruise down Commonwealth Avenue ("Comm Ave" to locals). My heart lifts as I relive being given my very own class.

It's another step away from financial services, another step into this unknown world. It's humbling to start over, to be an unpaid intern…and now a paid, real teacher with one of the worst timeslots (still practically an unpaid intern). I'd forgotten how hard it is to be back at the starting gate. But it's better to be at the starting gate of a more-promising path, than pounding down the furlongs of a race I didn't belong in. Yes, the corporate world would always offer more financial security and there was, excuse the pun, real *value* in that, especially for a kid who grew up poor. But financial security was no longer enough.

At the age of 49, my mother received the news that she had less than six months to live. I was now 31; 49 suddenly seemed terrifyingly close. Her life had seemed, to me, to be spent primarily struggling to make ends meet and raising us kids. The lesson I had taken from it was to avoid crushing poverty at all costs. And I had soldiered forth in that mission since I was 18 when I started working my way through college. But now it occurs to me that her too-early death held an even more important lesson in it: to live the happiest life you possibly can every single day. Because you never know if you're going to find out that you only have six months to live.

I'd spent years chasing financial security, but I wasn't happy. I wasn't making a difference. I didn't care about what I did. My corporate career and lifestyle aren't what I'd choose if I only had six months to live. It was time to try something else.

I brake at a red light and look up as the huge trees along the avenue rustle. Anything seems possible on nights like this. Without even thinking, I'd accepted the Monday night class. My head hadn't gotten in the way. My heart knew the answer all along: I was going to teach yoga.

It isn't perfect. The students might be ungrateful and uninterested. The studio space isn't ideal and my timeslots are crap to say the least. But there is potential here. And I'm excited to accept the challenge.

My teaching and fledgling transition to the yoga world, chug along with little visible progress. I try to remember the yearly progression from winter to spring. Deeply miserable when it's cold, I basically try to hibernate in front of a space heater from Thanksgiving through April. I roam around in bulky layers, pale and bemoaning the weather. Too busy cursing the luck of marrying a native New Englander who swears he'll never move, I forget to notice how the days get a bit longer each day and the ground slowly thaws, until one day I'm thrilled it's not dark at 4:30 pm and not quite as freezing. I can only hope that someday soon, my teaching will follow suit and show signs of a thaw.

In terms of survival in the meantime, I commit to not letting the struggles of teaching burrow into my sense of self like that first class. If I want to stay sane, they can't be my yardstick of success. Intellectually, I know that if only for my own survival, I can't allow my self-worth to rest on the experiences or feedback of others—*any* others. But knowing something intellectually and living by it are two entirely different things.

Remembering the time and tedium it took for me to surmount my anxiety, I resolve to illuminate the path and then step aside. The work and the success will be each student's alone—just like Thea said.

On a random Monday night notable only for its sheer averageness, I walk in, braced for the usual battle. The class will race through their practice and resent me for reining them in. They'll throw alignment and caution to the wind for the sake of flashy poses and cheap gains. A wiser woman might let them have it. But if it takes ten lifetimes, I'm determined to keep these students grounded, working the micro-facets of alignment, and teaching the yoga of discipline and doing less.

Dreading their floppy apathy, I grit my teeth and try to smile as I begin the first sun salutation. For the benefit of the one newbie, I demonstrate when I'd usually just verbally guide. I sweep my arms up and slowly flow down. I peek at the class. And jerk to a stop, shocked. I'm actually *ahead* of them. The students are still transitioning to standing forward bend. They are...*gulp*...going just as mindfully and slowly as I've been asking them to for months. I'm so surprised, I almost fall out of the pose.

Ashley, a petite blond who I've come to know as the diligent one who shows up every week and attempts the real work of the practice, catches my eye and smiles knowingly. She knows they've got it. I smile back, my heart speeding up as I realize that they've *really* got it!

The rest of the class is practically magical as the room fills with the quiet grace of hard work, conscious awareness, and still minds. The students move slowly, with intention. Alignment is strong instead of compromised for the ego of achievement. I barely need to make adjustments. The students harness their own power, connect to their intentions, breathe, and dive deep within.

I'm so happy I don't know whether to cry or run around hugging each person. I want to punch my fist in the air and scream, "Yes, yes, yes! You've got it!" But instead, I just smile giddily and let the yoga work.

After class, I'm so delirious with the thrill of it that I get in the car, mistake reverse for drive, and promptly back straight into the garage wall. Otherwise, it would've been an utterly perfect night.

Chapter Twenty-Eight

And Then There Was OM

It's the last night of my yearlong *Seva* Rotation. I teach classes at three studios around Boston now. Having more experience means I'm only slightly consumed with anxiety before each class—a stark contrast to the nervousness that used to completely overtake me. Maybe my emotional and physical bodies have adjusted.

Wait. Did I just use the terms emotional and physical bodies? Holy crap! Am I becoming a real yogi?

Being slightly consumed with anxiety is fine. My last *Seva* class signifies the end of the internship and the last vestige of my training. This was my first venture into the teaching realm, my first students, and I want to go out on a high note. Okay, fine—I want more than just a high note—I want to end on a freaking unforgettable, "You changed my life, thank you for the best yoga class ever!" note. I'm looking for an, "And the award for best teaching in the novice category goes to…" note. I want confetti to rain from the sky. Students to fall to their knees and weep. The Earth to pause on its axis.

Wait. Was that last one just a smidge too much?

Okay, fine. Maybe I'm not as yogic as I thought—that sounded rather competitive and egocentric, the antithesis of yoga. Although the fact that I at least recognize that is rather yogic…so where does that leave me? Yogi or not? Aware of my downfalls but still prone to them? Which am I? Where do I belong? Oh for God's sake, shut up, you freak!

Thanks to my own work on the mat, now I can actually stop the mental chatter. And in its place there is…blissful silence. I'm grounded. My focus is on the students.

The class is full. About 30 people, mostly regulars, attend each week. My teaching this night is steady and confident. The majority of the students—experienced, familiar to me, and accustomed to a mindful slow-flow system by now—open themselves to the practice and respond. The room steeps in the deep peace of hard work and still minds. Grounded and relaxed, I patrol the rows calmly. I make assists on sometimes-sweaty students confidently. Strangely, I no longer fear other people's sweat. In fact, the whole sweat thing seems kind of silly in hindsight.

On the stage that is teaching, in the show starring me, titled, "Sara Teaches a Class: Please Judge Her," I'm at ease in the lead role. I recognize that I'm the Pied Piper now—I offer the path and am sure of my ability to lead. I can distance myself from the outcome of whether I'm followed.

In fact, I'm so at ease, that I feel free to be myself. Like *really* be myself. Even my silliest, most embarrassing self. I loosen the tightly held boundaries that I'd relentlessly maintained for so long in financial services. I'd initially believed I would also need them in my new role as a yoga teacher, but now I know better.

I notice I'm overusing the word "delicious," in that way that you get stuck on a random word and then can think *only* of that word—as in "take a slow *delicious* transition to *uttanasana*," or "feel the *delicious* lengthening through your right side." But I keep using it anyway because I no longer care about cramming myself into someone else's idea of what I should be.

For the first time, I'm not reading from pages of pre-scripted sequence notes. But in the throes of being note-less and unguarded, I end up uttering the freakishly weird, "Transitioning into pigeon…feel that opening at the back of your right hip. *Mmmm. Yeesss.* Pigeon is deeeeelicious."

There are a few giggles. I pause, wondering what's so funny, then turn on my instant-brain-replay. I burst out laughing at my verbal gaffe, but also feel the compulsion to defend myself—correct my mistake, reestablish order—as Thea's ironclad rules about maintaining strong boundaries and establishing myself as a serious teacher at the helm of this class swoop in. Everyone needs to know that I know what I'm doing. "What I meant is that pigeon *pose*, as it opens the piriformis muscle, should feel good. There should be no strain."

I wait a few beats. Then decide to throw order and self-consciousness to the wind. To hell with it. I'm not Thea. I don't need to maintain impenetrable boundaries and the illusion of perfection. I'm just a new teacher bumbling my way through this class and doing the best I can. I channel my best Julia Child impression and add, "Pigeon, braised in olive oil, then gently sautéed to a delicate finish, is quite delicious indeed." This time, the whole room erupts in laughter. We're a coordinated unit, all laughing at me and it's okay. In fact, I'm still maniacally entertained even after everyone else isn't.

Nunnally catches my eye and winks at me. I'm reminded that he once told me, "I love your laugh—it's so crazy and weird. You sound completely insane and maybe a little dangerous, but I think it's cute." Already aware of this, in part due to the sideways glances my natural laugh often elicits, I usually stifle it. But not tonight. It's liberating to not give a crap what anyone thinks—to fly my freak flag high with unadulterated pride.

Or, at least you know, at a still respectably weird half-mast.

I wink back at him. The mood in the room is buoyant, happy, calm. I gather myself, strike a more serious tone, and continue the class. The students plod on as if we'd never digressed. I'm not exactly sure what I feared would happen if the strictest boundaries slipped just a little, but chaos doesn't reign and students aren't psychologically scarred. Am I perhaps more approachable and human for letting them see this chink in my perfect class plan? Or does everyone just appreciate a moment of levity as they slog through the murk of themselves?

Whatever it is, it works. Mindful concentration reengages. Breath deepens. Students reconnect to their intentions and press forward. This journey is not yet complete.

As the class toils onward, a woman at the back lays down on her mat and starts laughing. Not in a giddy, "I've reached nirvana," way (if, indeed, that might happen). But in an, "I'm trying not to cry," kind of way. I make my way over and kneel next to her.

"I'm sorry. I swerved to avoid a bus on the way here and fell off my bike. My entire left side hurts." She pulls the long sleeve of her shirt up and there's blood running down her arm. She claps a hand over her eyes and tears slide under her fingers.

I don't know what I was expecting, but nearly getting hit by a bus wasn't it. "I'll be back with the first aid kit."

"Lifting the heart, take three cycles of *pranayama* here, stay with your breath...." Still verbally guiding the class, I walk to the closet and retrieve the kit. I bring the class into child's pose and quickly bandage her up. I'm so focused I forget to put latex gloves on first. "Why don't I help you into a restorative pose?" I suggest, closing the kit.

She nods, bringing both hands over her face. "Is everyone staring? I'm sorry. I'm so embarrassed. Did I get blood on your arm?"

She did, but the important thing is that she's okay. I look at her mat neighbors. They are politely, studiously, looking straight ahead. "Nobody's watching. I promise."

Still bringing the rest of the class through the sequence, I gently help the student into a restorative pose. I fold her sweatshirt and drape a sleeve over her eyes. Then, instinctively, I place my palms on either side of the makeshift eye pillow. I don't hesitate to touch her. My fears around touching people, germs, sweat, even *blood?* Gone. I wait a long moment. Then I leave her in privacy and return to the front. On my way, I pump an excessive amount of the hospital-grade hand sanitizer from the wall dispenser on my hands and up my arms. Nonetheless, I'm careful not to touch any other students.

She stays in the pose for the rest of class. Her body looks limp and relaxed. She doesn't even move for *savasana.* I end the practice and she's the last to stand. She bows over her hands and smiles at me, looking rested and peaceful. I bow and smile back.

Catching sight of the clock, I realize I'd been fully absorbed in every moment of the class. My brain hadn't wandered ahead or relived the past. Just like my first class as a student. I've come full circle. It feels great.

My regulars come up and sincerely thank me. My yoga dreams come true as they tell me that I was a fantastic teacher, that I have changed their practices and brightened their Sunday evenings. I'm humbled...grateful beyond words. Let's be honest, I'm even a bit giddy.

Ashley, the petite blond who'd become my first regular, touches my forearm. "I can't remember exactly what you said...something about letting go of something in our lives that no longer serves us and welcoming in something new...anyway I loved it. I felt like I worked so hard, like from the deepest part of myself. And I feel so great now, like cleansed or something. Anyway, I just wanted to say thank you and I'll miss you."

Ashley isn't the most flexible student in class. She isn't the tiniest, or the strongest, and she never even tries inversions. But Ashley is the most yogic because she always shows up. She works hard, tunes in to her body, and then lets each practice be only and exactly what it is. No matter how cold it is on a snowy New England night, or how gorgeous of a sunny summer day, or how busy, or tired, or congested she is, Ashley shows up, tunes in, and then lets go.

She looks a bit teary-eyed as she stands on her tiptoes to give me a hug (because after all, she's a person of average height and I'm a towering giantess). I'm a bit teary too.

As we walk out after class, Nunnally slings an arm around me. "I'm so proud of you," he says, kissing the top of my head. "You're an amazing teacher." He takes me out for a celebratory dinner and I ravenously inhale not just one, but two entrees at our favorite Thai place. Much later, we return home and I attack the house in what can only be described as a cleaning frenzy. (Because what else would I do?) But hours later, I lie, still awake in the wee hours, wired over the events of the evening.

As is my wont, I replay it. The class had been an unequivocal success. I'd tended to a vulnerable, injured student and allowed myself to be goofy and embarrassing in front of a roomful of people. For the first time, I'd been *utterly authentic* in a work setting. From my bare feet to my teaching, I'd been unsheathed. Myself. And that felt an awful lot like...yoga. Authenticity is, after all, the very essence of yoga. And it was a lack of authenticity that had fueled my exodus to yoga training in the first place.

I'd found no room for any expression of individuality in my corporate career. Within the financial blandscape, there was hardly any variation in skirt length or hair color, let alone a career path beyond the narrow confines of preestablished corporate margins. Clearly, I'd never fit in that restrictive world any better than I fit in its business suits.

Realizing on some level that I preferred bare feet and yoga mats to cubicles and high heels, I'd sought out teacher training as a form of escape. A source of oxygen. After all, I'd experienced an intoxicating blend of freedom, support, and release as a casual student, so surely I'd find the mothership of all that and more in a training. Surely, in a world where people were allowed to look and dress and live outside the lines, where indeed, being "outside the lines" was celebrated, the inhabitants would be accepting of all. Even accepting of a friendly and eager, though comparatively uptight, corporate refugee in her freshly laundered, unstained yoga gear. Even in spite of her lack of tattoos, piercings, or veganism.

But when I finally mustered the courage and entered Yogadom, I ran into some of the same snarky unkindness there. In between chanting and down-dogging over the knife in my back, many of my fellow trainees were too busy competing to show Thea who was the most yogic to actually *be* yogic. Which had revealed that there was just as much posturing in the yoga world, it was just disguised differently. *Total bummer.*

But now I wondered if perhaps I'd allowed the pendulum to swing too far from idealization to cynicism. In my disillusionment, I'd negligently lumped everyone into one of two categories: New-Age lunatics or faux yogis (faux-gies?). And while the latter certainly had proven its unfortunate existence, it was the former that I'd misjudged. Yogis who are genuine in their unique wackiness *do* exist. They've simply breathed and stretched and meditated themselves into a place where they're entirely comfortable being only themselves. Just as I'd breathed and stretched and meditated to where I was (fairly) comfortable being myself. And because of that, I now had a deeper connection, understanding, and perspective on myself and my relationship to the rest of my life, as well the larger world around me.

Originally, I'd been too caught up in my expectations and corporate-formed judgments (the very ones I was trying to escape!), to see that plain fact. But tonight I'd relinquished my tight hold on maintaining roles and the rules that go with them. I'd released trying to live up to some idea (my own, Thea's, or anyone else's) of what a "teacher" should be like. And it was that very letting go that had enabled me, for the first time in an official "work" setting, to be my most honest and real self.

My journey wasn't complete. But at least I'd found the right path to start down, and somewhere along it and in doing so, I'd already found my way hOMe.

Chapter Twenty-Nine
...But Now Am Found

Sometimes I think of Ashley and her parting words. And I remember a certain Tuesday night when I was a student in Thea's class, and I had thought of her as the Pied Piper as she had led us on a course to draw us into the deepest parts of ourselves. I'd marveled at Thea's incredible talent and thought how inadequate I was in comparison, how her turn of phrase was so brilliant, while I, meanwhile, could never think of what to say. How she had provided a spark that I'd fanned into a blaze of awareness, and, ultimately, liberation.

I could ask for nothing more than to provide a spark for one of my students. To pass onward the possibility of inward-gazing, meditative silence to someone else. I wasn't the creator of this possibility, I was merely a conduit, a tour guide, pointing out the path to melting into a deeply rejuvenating, exquisitely restorative, overall reconstructing of oneself. In doing so, I had become a stitch in the tapestry of time and tradition that stretched 7,000 miles east to India and 5,000 years passed to a time when yoga began. Or at least began to be recorded.

I submit that the most powerful action any of us can take is to brighten or enhance, improve or support, in effect, to *alter* (however subtly) another person's path. That there's no better way to indelibly mark your own place in the world than to stretch out your hand to someone else. And that to be part of another's journey, somehow, in some way, is the most meaningful contribution anyone can make.

I think of the teachers along my own journey, both within and beyond yoga: the tiny regal yoga queen who taught my first class and set me on the path; Thea, who swirled me up in a centrifuge, spinning apart segments of my identity and then plunged me down a rabbit hole where the path twisted and wove through conflicts and questions; Nana, with her tremendous spirit and generosity; and my aunt Joan, that innate yogini and dearest mentor whose never-ending support, wisdom, and love had guided and shaped me for as long as I could remember.

I think of how my life has expanded under their influences toward the distant prospect of my more-evolved, more-authentic self. In their own ways, all of my teachers had helped me as I inched across the chasm toward the person I suspected I could be but was too afraid to actually become. Just as one's practice on the mat progresses imperceptibly toward transformation, so too had my professional and personal paths evolved.

And while some faux-gies will try to imitate or distract with an onslaught of New-Age idioms, what yoga is really about is peeling back the layers, or *koshas,* and revealing the light of the naked nucleus of the self. It wasn't some grand, external exodus of going to live in the Himalayas—it was a subtle internal shift within the maze of my everyday city-dwelling life. It was the courage to be myself.

Yoga: traditionally translated as "to yoke." To harness. To unite. May I humbly add to that list, perhaps, also, to *bridge.* To bridge the expanse between the infinite and the now, the thorny tangles of daily life and the surrender to something at once much larger than oneself and yet also intrinsically within oneself. To learn and to teach. To work hard and rest fully. To explore that delicate balance between striving and resting…and to be equally comfortable in either state. To unify our practice on the mat with our practice off the mat. And to remember, *to always remember*, that the answers reside within ourselves and we need only to be still enough so as to hear their call, let their radiance shine forth, and to be brave enough to follow the illuminated path.

Acknowledgements:

In loving memory of my Nana, Ann Marie D'Angelo DiVello, whose lifelong courage, tremendous spirit, and generosity were beautiful and blessed additions to my life and my Auntie, Evelyn Rita D'Angelo Mudd, Nana's partner in crime, older sister, and sous chef. Thank you, gentle Auntie, for being my third grandmother.

Professional thanks to:

Andrea Finlay, editor, advisor, coach, for your tremendous wisdom, incredible insights, creative ideas, and understanding this book's essence at its very deepest.

Crystal Patriarch, my publicist, for her creative marketing strategies.

Danelle McCafferty, developmental editor, for editing in all directions.

Julie Metz, yogi and amazing cover designer.

Sweet Pauley, life coach and a yoga compass.

Wayne Elizabeth Parrish, copy and line editor, the best eagle eyes in the universe.

Personal thanks to:

Joanie: Innate yogini, Earth mother, dearest friend. I will always aspire to be like you.

Uncle Martin: Your kindness, generosity, and humor mean everything. You're like a father to me and I'm thankful every single day for you.

Leigh: Who got stuck in the revolving door but hopped the fence between friend and family. I love all our memories, adventures, and your wonderful, deep-down, completely infectious laugh. Thank you for slogging through each tiny decision and particle of life with me; and for remaining surprisingly patient as you did so. Thank you, too, for suggesting that I "start writing again" on the road trip home from Philly. I did!

Katelyn: Years of memories, two weddings, one trip through Australia and several to Kripalu. Thank you for your support and for sharing in my genetic indecisiveness.

Hanna: Beloved sister, sous chef, surprisingly talented editor. Thank you for your avid support every day in innumerable ways. I am so incredibly grateful for you.

Annie: Thank you for your endless support. Even when I'm totally out of line.

Jessica: I enrolled in teacher training and graduated with a wonderful friend! Thank you for being my fellow "normal yogi" (no-yo). Thank you for your understanding and support along these journeys, book and training. Your astute insights (Tri Dosha Yoga!), enthusiastic encouragement, and completely awesome sense of humor are so fabulous and deeply appreciated.

Allan Petersen: My critique partner who understood my vision and helped me refine it even though you don't read memoirs or chick-lit and have never done yoga.

Andrea: Thank you for offering to read my book and then actually doing so—and in record time! Thank you for all your hard work, thoughtful insights, and incredibly kind words. Most of all, thank you for understanding the message of this book so deeply and completely. What a lovely surprise to meet a kindred spirit in the process—and to have that kindred spirit be such an amazing editor.

Thank you to my friends in financial services—proof that good can come anywhere. Laurel, Kelly, Patti, Wayne Elizabeth, Stephanie, Jane, Deneen, Brooke, Ginny, and the few, but truly good, guys I worked with, most notably Angelo and SCDJ.

Thank you to my nonfinancial services friends: Diana, Mary Beth, Reb, and Sandy for your tremendous support, encouragement, and insights.

And of course, my greatest gratitude goes to Nunnally, my best friend, who knows me better than anyone and loves me anyway. You are always welcome in my classes. Snarfing over "sphincter" or not. ☺

CPSIA information can be obtained at www.ICGtesting.com
Printed in the USA
LVOW12s2243070314

376535LV00004B/313/P